Juicing

by Neo Monefa

Table of Contents

1. Welcome to the Wonderful World of Juicing

Do you often wake up in the morning with a sluggish feeling-- as if the whole world is weighing down on your shoulders? Does this lethargic feeling persist throughout the day leaving you without energy and drive to accomplish your goals?

You may have tons of paperwork piled up on your desk, a day's work of record keeping to do, or maybe a whole house that must be vacuumed, a mountain of laundry that need your attention, or a fun evening with your family that keeps getting pushed back into your calendar.

Does it already feel like a chore whenever you have to do anything proactive?

Well, if you answered "yes" to any of these questions, then you are one of many Americans who are feeling the same way. When you think about it, it's actually very simple-- such problems as those mentioned above can actually be attributed to one single thing: the lack of energy.

Now close your eyes and imagine waking up everyday your mind fresh, your senses alert and your body feeling great. You have such a positive feeling that you know you can take on whatever the days bring you!

Now didn't that feel great?

If just thinking about the potential of what you can achieve with proper diet and nutrition already makes you THAT excited, can you imagine what it would be like to have that kind of feeling all the time? To actually live that life?

Well if you picked up this book thinking about how juicing can help you be healthier, more energetic and enthusiastic about life in general, then congratulations. You just made a very important decision, one that can potentially change your life for the better. Welcome to the good life, welcome to the wonderful world of juicing!

2. Juicing: The Healthier Alternative

You may have heard about juicing through the local news, through your favorite celebrity who has suddenly become an avid juicing aficionado, through magazines, or through your friends, neighbors or co-workers all swearing by this latest craze. Regardless of the source of information from which you learned about juicing, it is highly likely that you picked up this book because you wanted to get substantial and detailed information about juicing before you try it.

Certainly, there is a science to it and we would like to help you understand what juicing is all about, how easy it is to incorporate it in your daily habits, and what you stand to gain by making the conscious decision to mind your health and get more out of life through juicing.

What is Juicing?

Now, to get on with the discussion, what exactly is "juicing?" How is it different from
"smoothing" or even just drinking a glass of natural fruit juice daily?

Simply put, "juicing" originally refers to the act of extracting the juice of out whole fresh fruits and raw, uncooked vegetables and then combining the juices into a drink, which is then taken cold anytime during the day. In the past, we were only used to drinking fresh juice- traditionally either orange or apple- straight out of the carton or a bottle. Whenever we choose to juice fruits and vegetables, we are actually extracting all the good stuff, leaving only the fibrous pulp and indigestible fiber, which can then be thrown away. What is now left is the pure, natural juice filled with nutrients. When we drink the juice, such nutrients, now available in larger quantities than if we ate the fruits or vegetables whole, can now be easily absorbed by the body.

Popular fruits for juicing include the iniquitous apples as well as berries, citrus, pineapples, cranberries, papaya, and melons, among others. Today, drinking juice is no longer restricted to fruits but now also includes a wide range of vegetables including kale, collard greens, wheatgrass, cucumber, cabbage, Swiss chard, leaf lettuce, beets, celery, sweet potato, carrots, broccoli, fennel, kohlrabi greens, and even radishes, to name a few.

In juicing, extracting the juice is typically achieved with the help of high-powered extractors or juicers. Since juicing essentially involves transforming whole fruits and vegetables into liquid, you need an efficient juice extractor or juicer to do the job. Juicing machines for home use typically cost in the range of $40 dollars to over $300 dollars.

What the juicer does is to chop or slice the fruits and vegetables into tiny manageable pieces and then spin these around and around in such a way that the pulp or fiber gets separated from the juice. The pulpy remains are led to a special compartment, while the juice flows out, ready to fill your glass.

If you have no idea where to buy the best juicer or what factors to consider when buying one, the next chapter will help you out. For now, let us focus on juicing and its many benefits.

The Rising Popularity of Juicing

In the past, a small number of devotees have already cultivated a lifestyle that revolves around juicing. However, its popularity surged in the past two years mainly due to the endorsement of popular celebrities, such as Gwyneth Paltrow, Chelsea Handler, Nicole Richie, Alicia Silverstone, Reese Witherspoon, Kim Cattrall, and Blake Lively, to name just a few. These gorgeous, sexy women of all ages have all been spotted toting their favorite "blends" while out in public. Now if you thought juicing is just for women celebrities, you may be surprised to know that even heartthrobs such as Colin Farrell, Owen Wilson, and Edward Norton have also embraced juicing. Considering that both male and female celebrities have come to enjoy the benefits of juicing, then there is pretty good reason why it has become popular among these health conscious individuals. One way of telling when something has become so popular, and probably addicting, is when even large chain outlets such as Starbucks also begin selling their own healthy blends.

Juicing is also currently making its presence known in the healthy foods market. In fact, the global juices industry has posted annual increase in sales, and with the industry's growth, the annual sales figure is expected to increase by up to $10.7 billion by 2016.

Although the demand for bottled juice blends compete with other beverages, such as bottled water as well as sports and energy drinks, the thirst for juicing has continued to increase in the last few years. This is mainly due to the increasing demand for healthier alternatives, resulting from heightened awareness for healthy living.

Another indicator that juicing has become very popular these days is that, according to statistics, there has been a 60% increase in the number of juicers being sold in the market for last year alone. What this means is that more and more people are realizing the potential of juicing, not just as a trend, but as an honest to goodness way to keep them healthy and fit.

Smoothing, Juicing, What's in a Name?

By now, you may already be familiar about what juicing is and what the juice is supposed to look like when properly executed. However, one question may still be bothering you at this point.

So now we come to the million dollar question: Is Smoothing the Same as Juicing?

The answer is "No."

To compare the two, juicing is different from smoothing in that the former uses only the juice while the latter uses all parts of the fruits and vegetables being processed.

In juicing, only the extracted juices of the chosen fruits and vegetables are used and turned into a refreshing drink. This can be achieved in two ways. When using a masticating juicer, the machine masticates or grinds the fruits and vegetables down. As it does so, the juice is slowly extracted and the remaining material is discarded. The final product is a thin, watery liquid that packs all the nutrients from the masticated fruits and vegetables into a few ounces of liquid.

Another kind of juicer, the centrifugal juicer, spins the ground bits of fruits and vegetables. The centrifugal force then separates the liquid from the pulp. The juicer basically produces the same final product, the liquid components of the processes fruits and vegetables.

One advantage of juicing compared with smoothing is that here, you get more of the essential nutrients packed into the liquid. If you are the type of person with a sensitive digestive system that cannot easily digest whole fruits and vegetables, then juicing is definitely the option for you.

Furthermore, removing the fiber from the fruits and vegetables, and ingesting only the good, liquid stuff means that the nutrients are quickly absorbed by your body. This is because fiber is the natural substance that helps the body slowly absorb nutrients from the food we eat.

In addition, you can consume "more" fruits and vegetables when you only drink the juice. However, others would say that the liquid is less filling than a blended smoothie.

In comparison, with smoothing, you dump your fruit and vegetable of choice onto a blender, and then whip everything up until you get a smoothie. Here, both the juice and the pulpy or fibrous parts of the fruits or vegetables are also included in the drink and then ingested.

Using a blender, you can create a final product that is creamier and thicker, simply because the fibers have been incorporated into the drink. However, a smoothie is more filling than juice. Thus, you may have to consume more fruits and vegetables before you can have the same amount of nutrients that you can find in the extracted juice alone.

What Can Juicing Do For You?

Certainly, one of the main reasons why juicing has become so popular these days is that it has so many health benefits and is so convenient to prepare. In a classic case of "Why didn't I think of that before?" many people are slowly becoming juicing devotees simply because the idea is so simple yet so ingenious. Who would have thought that there was actually a shortcut in enjoying all the health benefits of "eating" fruits and vegetables without exerting effort in cooking and preparing them?

In this part, we will discuss with you some of the most important advantages of juicing as a healthy alternative.

Perhaps to underscore what juicing can do to your body, you may liken the word "juicing" with "supercharging," because this is exactly what you are doing, you are supercharging your body by increasing nutrient intake through drinking pure vitamins, micronutrients, and even enzymes found in fruits and vegetables.

As you do so, you not only avoid the chemicals found in processed food, but also radically initiating wonderful changes in your body, such as boosting your metabolism and reducing or neutralizing your body's acidity levels.

- **Speaking of acidity, stress and even toxins found in our environment can make our bodies more acidic than it should be.** When this happens, our body becomes more conducive to acquiring diseases because our immune system is considerably weakened. However, with juicing, we can restore the normal acidity of our body, thus preventing diseases.

- **Juicing also promotes cell regeneration.** As previously mentioned, high acid levels in the body make it weaker, unable to perform healthy functions such as cell generation. In fact, cancers thrive in bodies that cannot properly regenerate cells. To avoid this, it is best to drink extracted liquid from fruits and vegetables such as beet, lemon, avocado, tomatoes, broccoli, carrots and berries, to name a few.

- **In relation to the above, juicing also prevents premature aging.** High acidity levels in the body increase oxidative stress that lead to age spots and wrinkles. With juicing, you can have fresher, more radiant skin.

- **Vegetables such as cauliflower, broccoli, kale and cabbage contain phtonutrients that include indole----3----carbinol (I3C) and diindolylmethane (DIM).** When you include these in your recipes, you will get the benefits of improved, blood sugar control, and reduced body fat. Hence, one of the most important benefits of juicing is that it helps with weight management.

- **Another major benefit of juicing is that it can help us maintain normal levels of blood pressure.** This is because our arteries become dilated when our body's acidity level is high. If this is the case, then it becomes difficult to control related symptoms of hypertension, arrhythmia, increased blood pressure, and even heart attack resulting from these.

- **Electrolytes, including sodium, calcium, potassium, and magnesium—the stuff found in most fruits and vegetables—help our body function well.** Without these, we may feel less energized and not get the full benefits of a well---functioning body. With juicing, you can increase your intake of fruits and vegetables that contain these electrolytes.

- **You may not know it, but fatty acids actually serve important roles in nerve and brain functioning.** When then metabolism of fatty acid is disturbed, you may be prone to potentially debilitating neurological diseases such as multiple sclerosis. With juicing, you can promote lipid and fatty acid metabolism in your body.

- **Once again, high acidity levels in our body may lead to a poorly functioning circulatory system, wherein there is "corrosion" in the veins, heart tissues and arteries.** This is because the acid in our body weakens the cell wall membranes that make up these tissues. With juicing, you can reduce or neutralize acidity levels in the body to help strengthen the circulatory system.

- **Finally, the normal cells become "sick" and unable to function properly when the body that houses them**

is acidic. Drinking the juice of fruits and vegetables that neutralize acidity can help you ensure that more oxygen is delivered to all cells in your body, thus promoting healthier cells.

Doing It The Right Way

With all the benefits listed above, you are probably super excited to try out this healthy alternative. After all, who wouldn't want to feel younger, fresher, have more energy and reduce risk for diseases with something so simple and inexpensive?

Here are some tips to ensure that you are "juicing" in a safe way.

- **Keep in mind that juicing is not a diet in and of itself— you still need to consume over 2000 calories per day so that you still have a balanced diet.** Although juicing can supercharge your body with much needed phytonutrients, your body still requires sufficient amounts of protein, fat, vitamins, carbohydrates and minerals that you will not necessarily get from just drinking the juice of fruits and vegetables.

- **It is best to drink freshly prepared juice every time.** This is because the juice that you prepare beforehand could develop bacteria once it's been exposed to various pathogens in the environment. Extracted juice that has been left to stand for too long may also have reduced nutritional value, not to mention the fact that it may have an unpleasant taste by then.

- **As mentioned earlier, in juicing, you only drink the liquid component of the fruits and vegetables, the fibrous, pulpy bits are always discarded.** Thus, you may also want to incorporate a small amount of fiber

into your diet just to make sure that your digestive
system is running well.

- **Finally, though it is pretty obvious, do wash the
  fruits and vegetables thoroughly before extracting
  their juice.** Washing them helps remove pesticides or
  dirt that may be present. At the same time, wash all
  utensils to be used (including knives, glasses and
  chopping board). Then, you should also clean the juicer
  after every use. The manufacturer usually provides
  cleaning instructions in the manual.

This opening chapter gave you an overview of juicing, its
definition and why it is different from smoothing. We also
explained the reasons behind its resurging
popularity and most of all, we listed down the many benefits
you can gain from juicing. The chapter ends with a few smart
tips to ensure that you are juicing safely.

The next chapter will be devoted to juicers— how to choose
the right one, the factors to
consider when choosing one, pricing guide, and so on.

3. Juicers Galore

This chapter is all about juicers. In particular, we shall show you the many different kinds of juicers in the market, factors you need to consider when choosing a juicer, some tips on how to maintain your juicer, and reviews of the top juicers being sold in the market right now. In other words, this chapter shall provide you with important juicer related information, which brings you closer to a healthier, more energetic lifestyle.

So, What Type of Juicer Should You Buy?

This seems to be the first question that pops up in anyone's mind when coming across the concept of juicing. It is possible that you are reading this book right now because you want to find out what kind of juicer you should buy. You may already have an idea about what kind of juicer you want. If you've seen those endless Jack LaLanne infomercials on TV, then there you go, that's a basic juicer.

However, there is no one perfect juicer out there. Just as there are many kinds of fruits and vegetables to mix together to create your own "blends," then there are also many types of juicers available in the market they differ in size, function, price, and so on. So, for a newbie, how do these juicers differ from one another? How do they compare?
How do you know which one suits your lifestyle? Let us answer these questions one by one, and we shall begin by identifying the basic types of juicers.

Masticating Juicers

Also known as "cold press juicers," masticating juicers derive their name from the word "masticate," which means to soften, crush, or grind food. Basically, masticating juicers produce juice by crushing and pressing fruit and vegetables. As in humans, a basic masticating juicer "chews" fruits and vegetable fibers, breaks them up and produces juice with greater yield. The juicer does this with sharp blades that first cut up the fruits and vegetables, before they are pressed down to extract juice from them.

The masticating juicer is the best choice for someone who really likes fresh juice, is into cleansing, and would also like to make other slow pressed food products with the masticating juicer. This type of juicer is also perfect for those who wish to extract the most minerals and nutrients from the fruits and vegetables that they process.

Advantages/Disadvantages of a Masticating Juicer

One of the most important advantages of a masticating juicer is that this type of juicer is more efficient than other types because they produce more juice from the same amount of fruits and vegetables than other juicers. Thus, for example, you get more apple juice from two apples from a masticating juicer than from a centrifugal juicer processing the same number of apples.

In addition, masticating juicers can extract juice from virtually all kinds of fruits and vegetables. In fact, some types of masticating juicers, such as the single gear juicers can even extract juice from traditionally difficult vegetables to extract, such as spinach, parsley, lettuce, wheatgrass, herbs, and other kinds of green and leafy vegetables.

Second, while extracting juice, masticating juicers do not produce greater amounts of heat and froth as much as the other types. Because it must operate at a slow speed compared with a centrifugal juicer (which has to run in high speed), a masticating juicer is capable of keeping nutrients from the fresh ingredients because of the moderate temperature they have during extraction. It is also for this reason why juice extracted through a masticating juicer has a longer shelf life, thus reducing wastage.

Third, masticating juicers can be used for other purposes such as making thick sauces, ice cream, sorbet, baby foods, and even nut milk or nut butter. Some of the more expensive ones can even help you make small bread sticks and pasta. In terms of disadvantage, masticating juicers work slowly and surely, hence, it may not be ideal for those who are on the go and want to extract juice quickly. Furthermore, masticating juicers also tend to be more on the expensive side compared with other juicers. However, we are sure that the advantages we have listed above far outweigh the disadvantage brought about by a more expensive price tag.

Centrifugal Juicers

Now let's go to the second type of juicer, which is the centrifugal juicer. If the masticating or slow press juicer is more on the expensive side, then the centrifugal juicer is more popular because it is more reasonably priced. The reason behind this is that it possesses one of the simplest mechanisms compared with other more complex juicers.

Centrifugal juicers employ a rapidly spinning blade that spins against a filter, which is responsible for separating fruit and vegetable juice from their original, pulpy, and fibrous state. From its name, we can tell that the centrifugal juicer utilizes centrifugal force to extract juice from your chosen fruits and vegetables. Centrifugal force refers to the force generated when something moves away from a center or an axis. In this case, the fruits and vegetables are sliced, ground to a pulp and then spun around so that the juice is separated from the juicy pulp. The juice drips down one chute, while the remaining pulpy fibers go down another chute.

Generally, centrifugal juicers come in designs that feature large chutes that can accommodate smallish fruits, such as apples and oranges. Thus, this is perfect for people on the go since you can save a few precious minutes of your time cutting and dicing the fruits and vegetables before you can juice them..

The centrifugal juicer is an excellent choice for those who don't have a lot of money to spend on the more efficient, but expensive masticating juicers. This is also ideal for people who don't mind getting fewer amounts of nutrients per processing as long as they are able to extract enough juice for drinking.

Did you know that a centrifugal juicer also works best for processing fruits ad vegetables for cooking and baking purposes? If, aside from juicing, you are also passionate about cooking and juicing, then the centrifugal juicer is the best choice.

Advantages/Disadvantages of a Centrifugal Juicer

As mentioned above, one of the advantages of using centrifugal juicers is that it can rapidly and quickly extract juice. Hence, this is the perfect choice for people just like you who may want to have their juice on the go. The centrifugal juicer is also perfect for extracting juice from tougher and harder parts of fruits and vegetables, such as pineapple cores, since a centrifugal juicer features steel blades that cut and slice fruits ad vegetables before the juice is extracted.

Another advantage is that centrifugal juicers are less expensive than their more complex, high end counterparts such as the masticating or slow press juicers. Thus, if you are a newbie juicer and want to experiments for the first few months, then buying a starter centrifugal juicer is the perfect, commitment free way to get started.

Yet another advantage is the fact that you can use your centrifugal juicer to process other ingredients for cooking and baking purposes. Hence, buying a centrifugal juicer is actually like buying two or three machines for the price of one!

In terms of disadvantages, one concern lies in the fact that the rapidly spinning action that is responsible for separating juice from the pulp is the same action that generates excess heat. Such heat can reduce or kill the enzymes from the juice you are producing. Hence, the nutrient value of the final product is lessened compared with what you get with a masticating juicer.

Meanwhile, centrifugal juicers may also produce less liquid ounce of juice from your chosen fruits and vegetables compared with masticating juicers. This is because the high speed, rotation is not efficient enough to extract 100% of the liquid from the fruits and vegetables. In fact, the pulpy byproduct of the centrifugal juicer is still moist, proof that not all of the liquid is separated from the pulp.

In addition, while a centrifugal juicer can also be used to extract juice from green leafy vegetables. However, the yield is considerably less than that of the masticating juicer.

Finally, when using a centrifugal juicer, the shelf life of the final product may also be shorter because juice extracted from this type of juicer tends to have more oxygen in it. Since the very basic operation of a centrifugal juicer requires high speed spinning action, this process aerates the liquid, incorporating oxygen into the final product. The generated oxygen bubbles lead to oxidation that, in turn, leads to quick spoilage of the juice.

Twin Gear Juicers

Finally, the last type of juicer we will feature here is the twin gear or triturating juicer. According to juicing experts, of all the juicers available in the market, this is the most efficient and has the best features. Of course, these come at a hefty price tag. Nevertheless, devotees believe that the expensive price of a twin gear juicer is outweighed by the many advantages you can get from this product.

How does it work exactly?

A twin gear juicer works in a similar way to the masticating juicer. Basically, it presses sliced fruits and vegetables using two interlocking gears that roll continuously, hence the name "twin gear." The difference with the masticating juicer, however, is that the twin gear juicer works at an even slower speed than the masticating juicer.

With a super slow speed, the twin gear juicer is capable of breaking open even the tougher cell walls, thus releasing more nutrients, enzymes, vitamins, and minerals from whatever it is you are juicing.

A twin gear juicer is also called the "triturating juicer." Literally, "trituration" refers to the process of crushing or grinding food into ultra fine particles. Hence, what the triturating juicer or twin gear juicer does is to crush and grind fruits and vegetables intro extremely fine particles so that everything is turned into juice.

Juicing experts believe the basic features of the twin gear juicer comprise its many advantages. For instance, the twin gear juicer can extract juice of very high quality, it operates at low speed thus producing less noise, it can be used for purposes other than juicing, and , it can produce greater yield per fruit or vegetable,

With the latter feature mentioned above, you can tell that the twin gear juicer is more efficient because the pulpy byproduct it produces as it separates the liquid from the fibers is the driest of all, in comparison with the byproducts generated by the masticating juicer or by the centrifugal juicer.

If these reasons do not convince you of the superior juicing power of the twin gear juicer, then do read on as we present the other advantages of the twin gear juicer in the next segment of this chapter.

Advantages/Disadvantages of a Twin Gear Juicer

As mentioned above, the twin gear juicer has so many advantages, let's take a look at some of them.

First, the twin gear juicer is considered the most efficient of all types of juicer because it is capable of producing more liquid ounce of juice from a variety of fruits and vegetables compared with a masticating juicer or a centrifugal juicer. The twin gear juicer is capable of extracting precious liquid even from small or tough leafy vegetables such as the popular wheatgrass, kale, spinach, pine needles, and a whole lot of other herbs and vegetables.

Second, it is relatively easier to use a twin gear juicer because it has a self feeding action, which sucks in soft fruits and leafy vegetables. This self feeding action is due to the twin gears that roll inward while crushing the fruits and vegetables fed into it. In case you need to juice relatively tougher produce, such as carrots, radishes, or even apples, you may need to slice them up into smaller, thinner, and more manageable parts.

Third, a twin gear juicer turns at a slower speed than the masticating juicer or centrifugal juicer. Thus, there is less aeration or incorporation of oxygen into the final liquid product. What this means is that you can store your juice longer for up to 36 hours because the juice will not spoil easily. The slow speed of the two gear juicer also means that it generates less heat than other types of juicers. Thus, you get maximum amounts of nutrients, enzymes, and other good stuff from your fruits and vegetables.

Fourth, as mentioned before, a twin gear juicer can be used for other purposes, making it an excellent investment in the kitchen. For example, it can be used to easily grind and crush tough produce such as apples, pumpkins and carrots, as well as easily crush soft ingredients at the same time. Thus, you can use your twin gear juicer not just to extract high quality juice, you can also use it for making baby food, ice cream, butter, sorbet, and even pasta and bread.

Finally, a twin gear juicer is a heavy duty machine. What you lose in counter top space, you gain in terms of performance, stability and durability.

In terms of disadvantages, the first obvious disadvantage is that it is quite pricey, with prices ranging anywhere from $500 to $1,000. It is also a bit more complex than a masticating juicer or the relatively simpler centrifugal juicer, hence, it is not ideal for beginner juicers.

Finally, there may be a considerable prep time involved in extracting tough produce since you will need to slice them so that they can easily be fed into the chute. If you are the type who want to have their juice fast, fresh, and easy then the twin gear juicer may not be the best option for you.

Some Factors You Need To Consider When Choosing A Juicer

As with other major purchases, you need to consider several important factors that can help you buy the right product. In this case, before you go out and buy a juicer, it would be a great idea if you knew about their basic features and operations. This is because varied types of juicers can also influence many things, such as what kinds of fruits and vegetables you can juice, how much juice you can produce, how fresh the juice can last, and so on.

In this part of the chapter, we shall break down this important decision into several key factors that you need to look into. As you go through the list, do keep your preferences in mind so that, hopefully, by the end of the segment, you would have already made the right choice. Then you can hop on over to our reviews to see if any of those juicers suit you.

Your Juicing Program

The first factor you need to consider before buying a juicer is your overall juicing program. Here, you need to ask yourself a few questions:

- Are you a beginner or an expert?

- Are you just experimenting or willing to make a commitment to the juicing lifestyle?

- What kinds of juicing blends are you going to try?

- Are you only going to use it for fruits only, for vegetables only, or for both?

Depending on your answers to the questions above, then you will be able to narrow down your choices and ultimately select the best juicer that suits your needs and your lifestyle. First of all, are you a beginner or an expert juicer? Perhaps more readers belong to the first category, which why you are reading this book in the first place. If you are a beginner, then you may want to buy a simple, no frills machine that can do the job quickly and efficiently.

Second, if you are a beginner, then it is highly likely that you are still in the experimenting stage. What this means is that you have not yet established a preference for fruits only, vegetables only or a juice that combines both. If you are not yet sure of your preferences then it may be better not to invest a huge amount if money on a more expensive juicer only to find that you don't have the time to operate it or the patience to clean its many parts.

However, if you are bent on going all out, and plan to use the juicer to extract juice from virtually all kinds of fruits and vegetables, while gaining maximum yield and efficiency.

Ease of Use

In relation to the items mentioned above, ease of use is another important
consideration. Here, you may need to ask yourself a few more questions before making that final decision.

- Do you prefer ease of use or efficiency?

- Does your schedule allow you to indulge in slow press juicers or not?

- Do you prefer a juicer that is easy to clean and operate?

- Do you prefer a simple machine or a complex one?

If you are the type of person who is on the go and wants to have her juice fast, fresh and quick, then you may want to consider getting a centrifugal user. This is because the centrifugal juicer allows you to extract juice in mere seconds! Unlike the slower masticating juicer or triturating juicer, which operate on a slower speed, you can immediately get fresh juice with a centrifugal juicer in no time.

In terms of features, a centrifugal juicer also has a simpler design that uses fewer components. In comparison, the two other slow press types of juicers have more parts and more complex designs that a new user may find bewildering. Furthermore, a more complex design means more parts to clean and maintain. Hence, a very busy person may not appreciate a masticating or twin gear juicer.

Price and Cost Consideration

Last but not least in our list of major factors to consider is, of course, the price factor. It is not easy to spend hard earned money on something you are not 100% sure of. Thus, before setting out to buy any kind of juicer especially the more expensive ones, you may need to answer the following questions:

- What is your budget?

- Do you want to maximize the nutrients from fruits and vegetables using a high end juicer or are you willing to sacrifice this for a less expensive juicer?

First of all, it's your budget that is going to dictate what kind of juicer to get. Juicers range from a few hundred to a few thousand dollars. Which one should you get depends on your budget.

Usually, the more efficient slow press juicers, such as the masticating juicer and the twin gear juicer, are more efficient and have many parts that help maximize the amount of juice produced per extraction. These kinds of juicers usually have more complex operations, more parts, sturdier materials and are, therefore, more expensive. On the one hand, if you are ready to commit to a juicing lifestyle and if money is not a consideration, then we would suggest that you go all out and buy the more expensive but efficient juicers out there.

On the other hand, if your budget is limited and you are looking for something that is easier to use, has a simpler mechanism, and not to difficult to maintain, then you can go for the less expensive alternatives that still have the capability to juice with mid level efficiency, but guarantee fresh juice in mere seconds.

4. Preparing to Juice

In Chapter 3, we will now get deeper into the world of juicing as, this time, we will be discussing several things that pertain to the process of juicing itself, including the selection of the rights combinations of fruits and vegetables, health considerations, ensuring balanced flavor, preparation and storage, as well as other practical tips

Choosing the Right Fruits and Vegetables

First of all, juicing is supposed to be seamlessly incorporated into your existing diet habits and preferences. In other words, rather than totally overhaul your diet habits, juicing should enhance and improve what you have been doing so far.

There are two reasons why you need to carefully plan how you should introduce juicing into your diet program. Physiologically speaking, you don't want to shock your body by suddenly introducing rich and potent juice into your system on a regular basis. This shock may have detrimental rather than good effects on your body.

Psychologically speaking, you may already be accustomed to certain flavors, tastes, and textures in your preferred foods. The sudden introduction of juice that you may never have tasted before may condition your mind that it does not taste good, making it difficult for you to enjoy each glass of extracted juice. If it's not enjoyable, then what's the point right?

To help introduce juicing into your lifestyle, it would be better if you start with the proper selection of fruits and vegetables to juice. Depending on your preference, nutritional needs and discipline, you will be able to narrow down you selection to a few choice fruits and vegetables to incorporate into your diet. Here are a few tips to keep in mind.

Tip#1 - Start with something sweet.

It is important that you start off with sweet tasting fruits and vegetables. These include apples and carrots. Specifically, carrots are sweet enough to complement the bitterness of some fruits and vegetables while apples can also serve as the perfect base for when you decide to include more bitter leafy vegetables.

However, you must keep in mind that too much sugar or fructose in your juice can feed harmful yeast and other organisms that, in turn, lead to several problems. These include fatigue, excessive weight gain, upset stomach, and so on.

Tip#2 - Gradually incorporate vegetables.

So as not to shock your system as well as your taste buds, slowly incorporate vegetables once you have grown accustomed to drinking high powered juice everyday. As you use the more familiar carrots and apples as your juice base, you can then add vegetables gradually until you get used to the taste.

Although there is no doubt that green leafy vegetables, such as kale, lettuce and mustard greens, do wonders for your health. However, some people think their taste is not desirable, especially for newbie juicers. In order to get the healthy benefits of drinking extracted juice from these vegetables, mix them up with more familiar "tastes" that you already prefer. This helps you get accustomed to the flavor slowly until you become more comfortable drinking their juice.

Tip#3 - Keep this ratio in mind: 2-1-1.

Let's admit it, it can be very overwhelming trying to figure out what fruits and vegetables to juice, let alone determine the right amounts for each. To help you with this, perhaps this is a good number to start: 2-1-1. Consider it your code to unlocking the enjoyable and certainly healthy world of juicing!

Well, of course what we mean is as follows: 2 root vegetables, 1 leafy vegetable, 1 watery vegetable. For the root vegetables, try the small variants like carrots and beets to ensure a power punch of antioxidants to your drink. Carrots, of course, add sweetness to the final blend. If you want to add fruit, you can substitute it with apples or kiwis.

For the leafy vegetable, try to add 1 variant, such as broccoli, kale, collard greens, and so on. Then to add to the whole mix, you can add 1 water rich vegetable, such as cucumber or celery, to add vitamins into the mix and to ensure a smooth final product. You can then add mint or other herbs to make the drink more refreshing

Ensuring Balanced Flavor

As we have mentioned earlier, it is important to prepare and accustom yourself to the tastes and flavors of various combinations of fruits and vegetables. Juicing is not just about simply extracting juice from produce. This is also about being able to maximize the health benefits from juicing without sacrificing taste and flavor.

At the same time, finding the right balance of fruits and vegetables—in terms of variants and quantities—is not just a fun process, it will also ultimately determine whether juicing can become an integral part of your dietary habits.

Tip#1 - Choose the right sweeteners.

If you need to sweeten your juice but do not like to use carrots, then you can add apples instead. Specifically, Granny Smith apples are best for this purpose because they are not so sweet, a little bit sour, and better able to complement the flavors of extracted vegetable juice.

To balance the flavor, you can also add some lime or lemon juice so that the juice can also have a refreshing and cleansing function. The acidity of citrus juices can also induce healthy BM in the morning.

Tip#2 - Find the right formula.

As we have mentioned before, juicing is supposed to be a fun activity, not to mention a beneficial feature of anyone's diet program when properly followed. Some experts that a good juice contains some or all of the following flavors: sweetness, a tart taste, an earthy taste, a refreshing twist, and some hint of herbs and spices. Part of the fun of juicing is finding the right mix of flavors that you can incorporate into your juicing program. Here's a quick reference that you can use whenever you are looking for the right fruits and vegetables to provide you with the flavor you are looking for. Feel free to clip it and place it on your fridge.

Tip#3 - Don't be afraid to experiment.

As we have mentioned earlier, juicing should be fun! Thus, feel free to experiment on what tastes and flavors suit your taste. There is no bible as to what is the right combination to achieve the best nutrient content and flavor. At best, all we can offer are just suggestions. In the end, it's still up to you because it will be your body that's going to determine whether something is right or is not right for you.

Just remember, don't start right away with the heavy duty, hardcore juicing staples, such as kale, if you have not yet grown accustomed to its taste. There is nothing wrong with starting with familiar fruits and vegetables, such as apples, tomatoes, kiwis, and so on.

If the juice is a bit bitter, you can more apple slices; if the juice is too sweet, then add lime to give it an extra zing! Don't be afraid to experiment, this is the only way that you can find the perfect combination that suits you!

Juicing Your Way to a Healthy Body

You may very well be holding this book right now because you believe juicing is the best way by which to improve your health. You may also be interested in losing weight, and in this regard, juicing is also one of the best ways to achieve that goal.

In this part of the book, let us discuss related information as to how juicing can promote good health, increase your energy, maximize your nutrient intake, and help you manage your weight.

Fiber Is Still Good For You!

Another common mistake first time juicers make is that they think the fibrous byproduct of their juicers have no nutritive value. Hence, they often throw this away and not give it a second thought.

If you are thinking of the same thing, then you need to stop right there!

Studies have shown that even though an individual consumes extracted juice on a regular basis, he or she still needs to eat whole fruits and vegetables to maintain an ideal diet. A diet consisting of 100% juice, no matter how supercharged each glass is, is not a good diet.

In this way, even experts agree that people who juice still need to have fiber into their diet. One good way to reintroduce some fiber back into your diet, you can add a little bit of the fiber produced by your juicer into the juice you are drinking.

Preparation

In terms of the right way to prepare your juice, again, there is no standard universal way of preparing extracted juice. Aside from the strict rule of following your juicer instruction manual, all other things that are covered by preparation—peeling, cutting, washing, and so on—are entirely dependent on each person.

To peel or not to peel, that is the question. If you are unsure whether you need to peel something or not, then check your juicer manual. Some juicers cannot process the tough skin of some fruits and vegetables. If your juicer can handle it, and if you prefer keeping the skin (and the nutrients) intact, then make sure that the produce is organic and grown without pesticides. Certainly, there is a need to thoroughly wash the produce and the utensils you will be using when extracting juice. If you don't wash them thoroughly, the fruits and vegetables may still have pesticides, or worse, foreign bodies that can get into your juice. Washing also helps prevent bacterial contamination in your drink.

Storage and Other Tips

Once you have successfully extracted juice from your fruit and vegetable selection, you may find yourself asking the following questions: When should I drink the juice? Can I store it for a few hours or a few days? How shall I drink it—cold, warm, room temperature? If you too are asking the same questions, then check out the storage tips we have compiled:

- Ensure that your container can be sealed tight and does not have extra air space inside.

- Fresh, extracted juice is best consumed within 20 minutes after extraction. Depending on your juicer, however, you may be able to store juice longer from six hours after juicing (masticating juicers) to up to 48 hours in the fridge (twin gear juicers).

- The juice should be taken when it is at room temperature. Experts say that this is the optimal temperature by which you can drink it. If you have prepared and stored juice beforehand, you can take out the container and let it stand for a few minutes to even out the temperature before drinking it.

- Experts suggest that you swish the juice around in your mouth before gulping it down. As the juice mixes with your saliva, this process stimulates the digestion process, which is crucial to the body's ability to process the nutrients in the juice.

- It may be helpful if you drink your juice with an empty stomach. This way, your body can absorb the nutrients and all the good stuff found in your glass of extracted juice.

- In relation to the above, drink your most potent juices at the start of the day when you need a lot of complex carbohydrates to produce energy that you need for the day's tasks.

- Though some people believe that drinking acidic citrus juice in the morning may upset your stomach, this may not actually be true in most cases.

There you go! Some more important information you need to know, this time, in relation to the process of juicing itself. Let's see, we have already taught you all about juicers—what to choose, how to choose them, and how to check them. Then in this chapter, we taught you the basics of preparing your juice—from choosing the proper ingredients, ensuring flavor, tips on preparing and storing, and so on.

Congratulations, you are well on your way to being an expert juicer. So what's next then? Well, it's now time to buy the ingredients and check out recipes for juicing. The next chapter will help you navigate through this task. Are you ready? Let's move on to the next chapter and let's go shopping!

5. Let's Go Grocery Shopping

In this new chapter, we will be covering more specific aspects related to fruits and vegetables the two core components of juicing. Here, our goal is to share with you some useful knowledge, and of course, some practical tips specially related to shopping for produce, what you need to know before setting out to buy fruits and vegetables, some detailed health factors that you need to consider, and so on.

The Shopping List

By now, you must be very excited to get started with your juicing program. But before that, let us tackle the next important step before you can fully juice your way to good health. We are talking about shopping, of course! You cannot start your program if you don't have the fruits and vegetables—along with herbs and other produce—that you will need for your juice.

In this part of Chapter 4, we will share some tips on how to choose the right kinds of fruits and vegetables based on several key factors. Though it can be quite bewildering at first, being armed with the right kind of information will help you choose the right kinds of produce depending on your goal, thus helping you maximize your juicing experience.

What Do You Prefer?

First things first, you need to be able to identify your preference, which will guide you in choosing the right kinds of fruits and vegetables to put in your shopping cart. Regardless of whether you are an expert or new to the world of juicing, you will definitely develop your own set of preferences as you go along. If you have no idea where to start, do read on as we explain a few basic details to help you shop for produce.

Just as in eating food, juicing also follows one basic rule: go with what tastes good! Of course, this is a relative subject because what tastes good for some may not taste as good for the others. If you are new to juicing, it would be best to start with common fruits and vegetables, such as apples, carrots, citrus, and so on. Starting a juicing program with familiar tasting fruits and vegetables can help your body and your taste buds adapt to the new sensation of drinking extracted juice.

Later on, when you body grows accustomed to the taste of nutrient rich extracted juice, you can incorporate new stuff into your diet, such as green leafy vegetables, or juicing mainstays like cucumber, green snap beans, radishes, and squash, to name a few.

As you go along, keep a list of combinations that taste good and those that you body can accept (meaning you are able to drink their juice without adverse reactions). However, before concocting your recipes, it may be a good idea to consult your doctor first so that you can cross out fruits and vegetables that may contain elements that can be bad for your body.

Organic Vs. Non-Organic Produce

You may already be familiar with produce labeled as non organic and organic, with the main difference being the way such produce have been grown. Non organic produce are grown in the traditional way, meaning tons of pesticide, fungicides fertilizers, herbicides, soil conditioners, and the like have been used to grow them. Meanwhile, organic produce may be more expensive but these have been grown with little to no pesticide, thus ensuring higher and safer quality.

In contrast, organic farming uses sustainable and renewable techniques to encourage crop yield, preserve soil and water, and reduce negative environmental impact. These techniques include crop rotation and using mulch, compost, and other natural fertilizers and weed inhibitors to feed the soil and control bugs and insects.

For the purpose of juicing, it would be better if you buy organize produce simply because you want to prevent toxic those chemicals from getting into your juice. According to the Environmental Working Group, as you navigate your way through the produce section, keep in mind the so called Dirty Dozen and the Clean Fifteen produce. If, for some reason, you cannot buy organic produce in your area (maybe due to the lack of options, low budget, etc.), then avoid the Dirty Dozen. However, you can still safely consume the Clean Fifteen because they have been proven the have the least amount of pesticides.

Dirty Dozen: Apples, celery, strawberries, peaches, spinach, nectarines, grapes, bell peppers, potatoes, blueberries, lettuce, kale/collards

Clean Fifteen: Onions, corn, pineapples, avocado, asparagus, peas, mangoes, eggplant, cantaloupe, kiwi, cabbage, watermelon, sweet potatoes, grapefruit, mushrooms

Fruits and Vegetables to Aid Weight Management

Perhaps one of the top reasons why juicing has become so popular these days is that many women want to manage their weight, lose a few pounds, and gain a leaner body. If you have the same reasons, then you made the right choice. Juicing has been proven to aid weight management.

In fact, The Centers for Disease Control and Prevention provides a list of fruits and vegetables, which they recommend as part of a healthy weight loss diet routine. Below, let us take a look at some of the fruits and vegetables that have been proven to help people lose weight. Spinach, according to The American Council on Exercise, is a prime example of a healthy food that should be included in your diet program. Spinach is a low calorie but nutritious vegetable rich in iron, folate, magnesium, the powerful antioxidant known as Quercetin, as well as Vitamins A, C and K. People who love eating carbohydrate----rich fattening foods such as corn, rice or pasta, may substitute these with spinach, which only contains 7 calories per serving.

Watermelons are excellent fruits that you can include in your juicing program. Aside from their taste, they can help you lose weight because they are very filling while having low calories. In addition, the whitish portion of watermelon (the part between the skin and the red colored flesh, is rich in citrulline, an amino acid commonly found in sports drinks to help decrease muscle fatigue. Thus, by drinking watermelon juice, you can exercise for longer periods.

Grapefruits only contain around 40 calories apiece. Based on a study published in the ""Journal of Medicinal Food,"" compounds found in grapefruit improve your body"s ability to control blood glucose levels. In terms of weight loss, it has been shown that eating half a piece of grapefruit prior to every meal may help you lose up to a pound a week.

Furthermore, grapefruits contain a compound that improves tissue sensitivity to insulin, which in turn, assists in fat loss. Finally, similar to watermelons, grapefruits are also very filling (with a water content of at least 90%).

Artichokes are excellent staples of a diet program because they can help curb the appetite, similar to other water based fruits ad vegetables, without packing on the extra calories.

The Top Ten Fruits and Vegetables for Juicing

Now that you are familiar with some of the produce that you will need to start juicing. These fruits and vegetables, when combined, help us get the greatest amount of nutrients and the maximum benefits from our juicing program.

Indeed, according to Ashley Koff, a registered dietitian with celebrity clients, "What"s so wonderful about juicing is that it gives you the opportunity to introduce foods into your diet you wouldn"t normally eat."

With this in mind, let us take a look at the Top 10 popular fruits and vegetables meant for juicing.

• Carrots. Rich in beta carotene; excellent base that can mask the strong taste of green leafy vegetables such as kale
• Kale. Rich in iron and folate
• Wheatgrass. Rich in Vitamins C, E, and K; has high cellulose content
• Celery. Rich in potassium in your diet; has high water content
• Cucumber. Cool and refreshing; neutralizes the taste of vegetables with stronger flavors
• Pineapples. Contains bromelain, which can aid digestion
• Apples. Rich in antioxidants
• Cabbage. Rich in Vitamin C and folate; high water content
• Beets. Rich in beta----carotene, antioxidants such as lutein and zeaxanthin, calcium, and iron
• Lemon. Rich in Vitamin C; can neutralize acidity in the body

Apart from the abovementioned fruits and vegetables, Koff states that we can also add other "elements" into the mix to improve taste and nutritional value. Says Koff, ""Freshly ground flax seeds, avocado, almond milk, coconut milk, tahini, or walnut oil could be tasty ways to add a little healthy fat to your juice."

Generally speaking, fruits and vegetables serve as excellent sources of a wide variety of various nutrients such as folate, potassium, vitamins and so on. With juicing, you can also help reduce, minimize or even completely avoid risks of various diseases such as cancers, type 2 diabetes, stroke, cardiovascular disease, and so on. Furthermore, vegetables rich in potassium can also help prevent bone loss and the formation of kidney stones.

Fruits and Vegetables to Aid Weight Management

Perhaps one of the top reasons why juicing has become so popular these days is that many women want to manage their weight, lose a few pounds, and gain a leaner body. If you have the same reasons, then you made the right choice. Juicing has been proven to aid weight management.

In fact, The Centers for Disease Control and Prevention provides a list of fruits and vegetables, which they recommend as part of a healthy weight loss diet routine. Below, let us take a look at some of the fruits and vegetables that have been proven to help people lose weight. **Spinach** is a prime example of a healthy food that should be included in your diet program. Spinach is a low calorie but nutritious vegetable rich in iron, folate, magnesium, the powerful antioxidant known as Quercetin, as well as Vitamins A, C and K. People who love eating carbohydrate rich fattening foods such as corn, rice or pasta, may substitute these with spinach, which only contains 7 calories per serving.

Watermelons are excellent fruits that you can include in your juicing program. Aside from their taste, they can help you lose weight because they are very filling while having low calories. In addition, the whitish portion of watermelon (the part between the skin and the red colored flesh, is rich in citrulline, an amino acid commonly found in sports drinks to help decrease muscle fatigue. Thus, by drinking watermelon juice, you can exercise for longer periods.

Grapefruits only contain around 40 calories apiece. Compounds found in grapefruit improve your body's ability to control blood glucose levels. In terms of weight loss, it has been shown that eating half a piece of grapefruit prior to every meal may help you lose up to a pound a week.

Furthermore, grapefruits contain a compound that improves tissue sensitivity to insulin, which in turn, assists in fat loss. Finally, similar to watermelons, grapefruits are also very filling (with a water content of at least 90%).

Artichokes are excellent staples of a diet program because they can help curb the appetite, similar to other water based fruits ad vegetables, without packing on the extra calories.

Fruits and Vegetables to Avoid

Although juice can be extracted from most fruits and vegetables, there are some that are considered "unjuiceable." These fruits and vegetables are probably best consumed whole or raw, rather than being juiced.

First in the list is the avocado, which turns oily, mushy and superosft fruit that yields little to no juice. As a new juicing devotee, maybe you should just stick to guacamoles for now. Second is another obvious fruit, which is just as mushy as an avocado. We are talking about non other than a banana. Because they have little water content, they are simply not ideal for juicing.

Third is the less popular winter squash it is so tough, difficult to slice, and has little water content to yield a reasonable amount of extracted juice. The tough exterior may even damage less sturdy juicers, so it's best to stray from this vegetable altogether.

Fourth in the list are eggplants. Similar to a banana, an eggplant will not yield any reasonable amount of juice and will only turn super mushy and unusable when processed through a juicer.

Finally, we have rhubarbs. These have tough outer layers that can damage the slicers of centrifugal juicers or the blades of masticating or twin gear juicers. Beyond difficulty in preparation, rhubarbs also have high amounts of oxalic acid, which binds with the calcium in your body, rendering it useless.

Quick Shopping Tips

We have now basically presented an overview of what you should (should not) include in your shopping cart. Having gone through the previous sections of this chapter, you may have already created a list in mind as to what you should buy on your next shopping trip.

Now, let us give some important tips about shopping itself. As a novice fan of juicing, you may have or have not yet experience shopping for more produce in a conscious and selective manner. To help you survive this experience, here are a few shopping tips for you!

Tip#1. It would be better if you make a detailed shopping list before you leave the house. This way, you can buy everything you need faster. As you make your list, you can go back to the early sections of this chapter so that you can identify what fruits and vegetables you want to try out first.

Tip#2. As you make your list, it would also be ideal if you conduct a little online research as to what fruits and vegetables are in season. Buying in season produce guarantees that you get them fresh and at a lower price.

Tip#3. Remember the Dirty Dozen and the Clean Fifteen? Do keep these in mind as well while you are finalizing your shopping list. Remember, the Dirty Dozen are the produce that you should buy as organic produce while the Clena Fifteen are produce that are safe enough for consumption even if they are not organic.

Tip#4. Do bring a recyclable shopping bag. This is way better than using plastic bags.

Tip#5. Look for produce that has smooth, bruise free skin. Whether you are buying organic or non organic produce, anything that may have bruises or damage on the skin or the outer parts may indicate that it is no longer fresh or it has been mishandled.

Tip#6. Do mind the price. Although you need more produce for your juicing needs, you don't have to buy everything in bulk. Moreover, check whether the price indicated is per unit or per kg. If the produce is priced according to weight, then only buy what you need. However, if the produce is priced per unit, then go buy the largest or heaviest one you can find.

Tip#7. If you need to buy portions of, let's say, watermelons or green leafy vegetables, make sure that you buy those that have been bagged properly and surrounded by ice. You don't want to juice fruits or greens that are not fresh. Aside from bruising, you can also smell the produce as a quick way of checking freshness.

Tip#8. Finally, ensure that the produce you have bought are packed and stored properly.

Juicing Mistakes and How to Avoid Them

Finally, you have already bought your juicer as well as selected and bought the fruits and vegetables you want to try. Before making your first glass of juice, we would like to leave you with a word of warning by listing down some common juicing mistakes.

Armed with such information, you can increase the likelihood that your first attempt will be a success. The success of your entire juicing program may ultimately rest on how good (or bad) your first glass of extracted juice tastes like and if your body accepts it well without adverse reaction. To ensure success, here are some of the more common juicing mistakes and how you can avoid them.

Mistake #1 - Using too much sweeteners.

As we have explained earlier, while it is a good idea to start off with sweet, familiar tasting fruits and vegetables, do avoid relying too much on these sweeteners. This is because too much sugar or fructose in your juice can feed harmful yeast and other organisms that can lead to excessive weight gain, fatigue, upset stomach, and so on.

Mistake #2 - Drinking juice on a full stomach.

Even some of the diehard juicers don't know this: extracted juice should only be taken with an empty stomach. The reason for this is pretty simple: drinking your juice on an empty stomach is the only way by which the nutrients, vitamins, and minerals will go straight to your bloodstream. If you forgot about it, you may want to wait two hours after eating a full meal before you can drink your juice.

Mistake #3 - Treating juice as a meal in itself.

This is a dangerous misconception about juicing. Juicing is only meant to supplement your regular food intake, and not replace it completely. Although extracted juice from fruits and vegetables are supercharged with nutrients, it cannot replace the other good stuff you can get from eating other kinds of food.

Mistake #4 - Not drinking the juice immediately after extraction.

Although juice can be stored for up to two days (only when you are using a high end twin gear juicer), the best time to drink extracted juice is immediately after extraction. This is because the nutritional value becomes reduced the longer the juice sits. As we have mentioned earlier, fresh, extracted juice is best consumed within 20 minutes after extraction.

Furthermore, the extracted juice should be consumed at room temperature. This is because room temperature is the optimal temperature in which you can drink your juice. If you have prepared your juice beforehand, take out the container and let it stand for a few minutes before drinking it.

Mistake #5 - Not consuming juice properly.

It may sound surprising but did you know that you actually have to "chew" the juice before gulping it down. Here, "chewing" is not to be taken literally. In the world of juicing, "chewing" the juice means swishing the juice around in your mouth before gulping it down. The explanation for this is quite simple: as the juice mixes with your saliva, this process stimulates the digestion process, which is crucial to the body's ability to process the nutrients in the juice.

Mistake #6 - Using a dirty juicer.

For obvious reasons, it is a bad idea to use a dirty juicer in extracting a fresh glass if juice. For example, if you prepared juice in the morning, you need to clean your juicer thoroughly before using it again in the afternoon or in the evening. If you don't there may be issues with bacteria, buildup of debris within the small parts, and inefficiency of the juicer.

Mistake #7 - Using the same recipe over and over again.

Although you may eventually develop a preference for a certain combination of fruits and vegetables, it may be a bad idea to keep using that recipe over and over again. Aside from the obvious fact that your juice will taste blah if you keep using the same recipe, did you know that juicing the same green vegetables can actually lead to hormonal issues and build up of oxalic acid that may affect your thyroid gland. To avoid this, try experimenting on new blends. After all, variety is the spice of life!

In this chapter, we summarized specific nutrition related information about fruits and vegetables that you can include in your shopping list. We also gave you a list of some popular produce, a few quick tips on how to combine them depending on what you want to achieve, and some information about shopping for produce.

Finally, we have also given you a list of common juicing mistakes that you must avoid at all costs. Armed with such information, you can now try juicing and hopefully continue with this program until you achieve the desired results.

6. Juicing for Weight Loss

Benefits of Juicing

The next question is, is it more beneficial to consume extracted fruit or vegetable juice than to eat fresh and whole fruits and vegetables? The answer is a resounding yes. For one, the nutrients which go straight into our system make the body more efficient in performing its functions. Aside from this, there are also recent studies supporting the claim that juicing is healthier. Well, no one would find it difficult to agree with this. As we all know, the body needs to work when digesting the food that we eat. With juicing, the "work" that has to be performed when digesting foods can be used for other purposes.

Another great benefit of juicing is it allows our digestive system to have a break. This is important as the body can focus on other functions such as the healing process. That is why juicing is very helpful for people who are sick. They just have to juice the fruit or vegetable known to address a particular sickness. This is also very true when you have wounds or small cuts. The healing process is much faster if you include juicing as part of your medication. You can actually substitute juicing to over the counter medicines.

Another benefit, which women would surely love, is its crucial role in building metabolic processes. It also has a crucial role in the rebuilding and regenerating of healthy tissues that can make the body look more youthful.

Juicing also plays a significant role in various nutritional therapies. It is used in treating different illnesses and nutrient deficiencies. All in all, it has been proven that juicing is very effective in improving the well being and overall health of an individual.

Juicing for Weight Loss

There is no denying that juicing has numerous benefits that have become crucial not just in treating nutrient deficiencies and in improving body processes but also in our busy schedules. With the possibility of making nutritious juices in an instant, many women can surely address the nutritional needs of their family. More than that, they can now also have an effortless way of maintaining a healthy and youthful body. But if you think that is all juicing can offer, think again. Recently, it has been creating a buzz about its use for weight loss.

How can juicing aid in weight loss?

Anyone can surely lose weight by drinking fresh juice from fruits or vegetables as it helps in losing excess pounds. How does this happen? It aids in weight loss as it makes you calorie deficient. It brings about huge caloric deficiency because you only get to take in around 500 to 800 calories a day. So, the principle of juicing diet is achieving caloric scarcity by drinking juice on a daily basis. If you drink fresh juice daily, you can reduce calorie intake of up to 1,500 calories a day. This is equivalent to a weekly loss of about three pounds fat. The best thing about this diet is that it does not deprive you of energy. As a result, your metabolism will not crash and will help you realize an effortless and successful weight loss.

What's also great about drinking fresh juice is that it allows the body to absorb nutrients very easily. In this way, your body gets enough nourishment without having to take foods rich in carbohydrates and fats. This results to the easy flushing out of cholesterol. Another important thing is it does not create energy from the utilization of muscle tissues. With this, you can definitely maintain your sexy figure.

What are the benefits of juicing for weight loss?

Today, not everyone is already convinced about the effectiveness of juicing in losing weight. For example, the Center for Disease Control and Prevention has stated that there may be a connection between fresh fruit or vegetable juice intake and weight loss. However, they have also stated that fresh juice from fruits and vegetables have significantly low calories. It also makes you fell full after drinking, which helps you to avoid eating foods with higher calorie such as chips and chocolates.

With these, juicing has definitely become a popular way of losing weight nowadays. Consuming fresh fruit and vegetable juice has numerous advantages. Read on below to know more about these.

- **Fresh juice allows you to get all varieties of carbohydrates and complex vitamins.** This is practical as you don't have to worry about what kind of foods rich in carbohydrates to eat. It is also practical because you don't have to allot budget for other carbohydrates rich foods.

- **You also get a lot of antioxidants which have numerous benefits as well.** AS you know, antioxidants are known to help lower the risk of developing diseases that are lifestyle related. Examples of these are diabetes and heart disease. Moreover, antioxidants also help in preventing different types of cancer.

- **Fresh juice is the perfect alternative to your multivitamins pill.** You may not believe it but, yes, you can have fresh juice everyday and do away with your daily multivitamins intake. It is a perfect replacement as it is full of vitamins and minerals.

- **Drinking fresh juice also helps in cleansing your body.** In particular, it greatly helps in cleaning u your gut, which is essential in preventing colon cancer.

It also helps in the proper function of the different internal organs.

•   **You get all the benefits without any disadvantages or negative effects if you use organic fruits and vegetables.** With organic materials, you don't have to worry about pesticides and other harmful chemicals that huge agricultural crops companies use. As you know, chemicals that were taken by the body through consumption of foods can have a huge effect on the health of the individual. For women, it can affect the development of the fetus when they are pregnant.

•   **If you want an excellent snack, nothing can be better than fresh juice.** For one, it gives you all the nutrients you need without leaving you overstuffed. Another advantage is that it can give your diet the variety it needs.

•   **If you have hydration issues, drinking fresh juice can solve this.** Aside from the vitamins and minerals, fresh juice has water that can keep you hydrated.

•   **You can achieve your objective of losing weight by drinking fresh fruit and vegetable juice as it has high phytonutrients.** These nutrients are essential in supporting your body to have greater balance. So, if your diet has high phytonutrients, you can definitely lose weight in the time line you have set.

•   **You can do away with your purely carbohydrate or meat protein diet.** With fresh juice, you can have a wider option in terms of vitamin choice.

•   **You get the maximum nutritional value from fresh juice as you juice raw fruits and vegetables.**

On the other hand, the commercial drinks contain a lot of preservatives which are known to cause negative side effects in your health. With this, fresh juice becomes more preferred than commercial juice by more and more health conscious women.

• **The dissolved fiber helps in maintaining the level of cholesterol in our body.** AS you consume fresh juice, the fiber it contains gets dissolved in your intestines and bloodstream later on. This makes it perfect for individuals with cholesterol level problems.

• **Many think that fresh juice is not palatable.** Well, they are wrong. You can actually create more palatable and tasty fresh juice as you can create one using different fruits and vegetables. You can actually create your own juice recipe. Moreover, you can create a recipe that can very well address the nutrients your body is deficient of.

• **Fresh juice is cheaper and better.** This is because there are many wonderful and flavorsome recipes of fresh fruits and vegetables that you can try. With this, you can have so many options even if you are on a tight budget. We mothers will surely be happy about this as we always face the difficulty of budgeting money for house expenses.

• **A lot of mothers face the problem of their children lacking appetite during mornings.** As mothers we are always concerned about the health of our children. That is why we buy multivitamins that can help them have more appetite. With juicing, this can be addressed with spending money on multivitamins. Fresh juice can be a perfect breakfast for anyone and can greatly help in improving the appetite.

• **For people that really want to target the lowering of their cholesterol level, they can follow a**

juicing diet program with fruits and vegetables that target cholesterol. Fresh juice is very effective as it has no saturated fats or added sodium.

• **Another great thing about juicing is that you can have fresh juice whenever you want.** This means that juicing is flexible with your time particularly with your very busy schedule. Career women would find it very helpful.

• **For people who have addiction to caffeine, carbohydrate, fat or alcohol, juicing is the solution.** Drinking of fresh juice can help them stay away from these addictions. As we know, being addicted to these unhealthy food elements is harmful to our health. These are the ones that cause diseases and cancer. BY treating addiction fat, alcohol and carbohydrate, one would really lose weight as a result. Mothers can train their children to drink fresh juices in their early years. In this way, the children would less likely develop addiction to unhealthy foods.

For the longest time, pineapples have been known to help in losing weight. That is why there are numerous companies, with canned pineapples and pineapple juice as products that invest in TV advertisements to promote the benefits of pineapple particularly in weight loss. To know if this is true, read on below to have more knowledge.

Pineapple for Weight Loss

In general, fruits and vegetables have relatively lower calories than other food items such as processed and canned foods. For example, a slice of pineapple only has 40 calories. This is very lower as compared to biscuits or cookies that have more than 100 calories. So, even if you consume 2 slices of pineapple you won't gain weight as it has low caloric content. Another reason why it helps in losing weight id that it has no protein or fat content. It contains Vitamin C, Manganese, fiber and a lot of antioxidants that help people maintain a healthy body.

The water and fiber will help in filling you up. With this, you would not want to look for other unhealthy foods as you are already full. Having weak bones is another problem that many women suffer from. The Manganese from pineapple can help in strengthening bones. Eating too much makes you feel bloated. This definitely contributes to gaining a lot of weight if not prevented. This can be addressed by the Pectin present in pineapples. If coupled with Vitamin C, it helps you prevent bloating. Another great thing about pineapples is it has Bromelain, which is also known to help prevent the onset or development of cellulite. Bromelain also helps in promoting muscle elasticity and muscle strength.

With all these, one may assume that pineapples really do help in weight loss. However, do pineapples have special properties that greatly promote in weight loss? The answer is no. It can help but it can't really promote weight loss. Pineapples won't help you burn fat, which is a crucial part of losing weight. It definitely won't help in burning fat because it can't keep your blood sugar at a low level. It has a glycemic index that is relatively higher than other fruits.

The glycemic index (GI) refers to a numerical scale that is used to indicate how high and fast a certain food can raise blood sugar or blood glucose level. If a food has low GI, it will raise our blood sugar level in moderation. On the other hand, if a food has a high GI it may prompt a high rise in our blood sugar level, which is usually above the optimal level. This is unhealthy or undesirable as high blood sugar level worsens our cholesterol level, which is a factor why people gain so much weight. With these, it should be clear by now that pineapples don't really promote weight loss. It can help, so it would still be beneficial to include it in your diet.

You can use pineapples to replace your usual foods that have higher caloric content. However, you have to take note that you need to eat fresh pineapples and not the canned ones. Canned pineapples are loaded with sugar, which makes it really unhealthy. It also has lesser nutrient content as most of the nutrients are lost during processing.

Banana for Weight Loss

Another fruit that many people believe to promote weight loss is banana. Unlike pineapples, bananas have higher caloric content. A regular size has 108 calories and around 17.5 grams of carbohydrates. With these, there is also a myth that bananas are not good in weight loss diet programs as it has high calories and carbohydrates. However, it has low glycemic index equal to 51. With this, one might certainly think that it is really helpful in losing weight.

Whether it promotes weight loss or not, there is no denying that bananas are among the most nutritious foods. For one, it is dense with minerals and vitamins. It is rich in potassium, which is important in the regulation of blood pressure. It is also high in fiber and low in fat. These are essential in helping you feel full for a longer time. If this is achieved, you won't feel the need to eat a lot or frequently. As a result, you would lose weight.

The craze about bananas as great weight loss food has become even more talked about when the Morning Banana diet was developed by Hitoshi Watanabe. It even became more popular when Japanese opera singer Kumiko Mori announced that she lost a significant amount of weight in pounds. According to her, she lost 15 pounds in just a few weeks. During that time, it was a phenomenal weight loss diet among Japanese people as it is said to be the easiest and fastest way of losing weight. It became known around the world through magazine articles, TV shows, and word of mouth. The Watanabes have also written a book about the diet.

However, all these don't still answer the question whether bananas promote weight loss or not. Well, the answer is no.

Again, like pineapples, bananas don't help in the burning of fat. If fat is not burned, then you would not lose weight. However, it also helps in helping you lose weight if included in your diet program. Again, it does not promote but it can help in losing weight. According to food experts, bananas can help people lose weight if eaten in moderation. From this, it can be concluded that bananas don't really promote weight loss but can help if included in the diet program as snack.

Banana is a great food item as snack in your diet because it has potassium, which necessary in a low calorie diet. A low calorie diet with low potassium can lead to cardiovascular diseases, diarrhea, impaired cellular function and growth of muscles, and severe exhaustion. If you are planning to stick to a 1200 calorie diet, you can include a medium sized banana. This will account for 9% of your total daily calorie intake. In this way, eating bananas helps you become successful in your goal of losing weight.

By this time, it should be very clear that pineapples and bananas don't promote weight loss. These fruits only help you in losing weight. What needs to be considered is the amount of calorie you have to take daily. From this, you will base the amount or size of pineapple and banana you have to eat everyday or for certain days of the week.

Skin, Hair and Nails – Beauty Anti Aging

Aside from weight loss, beauty is another primary reason why more and more people are drinking fresh juice from fruits and vegetables. In particular, a lot of women are now into juicing because of its anti aging powers. When it comes to beauty, the skin, hair and nails are the first ones that we people see in a person. With this, we always adopt ways that can improve the health and glow of our skin, hair and nails.

Juicing for Healthy, Smooth and Glowing Skin

As women, we always want to stay beautiful. One way of achieving that is by having a glowing skin. Our skin glows if it is healthy from the inside. If we are following a healthy diet, it will reflect in the smoothness and glow of our skin. That is why many women are also patronizing skin care products. Millions of women use numerous skin products such as lotion, moisturizer, cream, body scrubs and many others. However, many of these products have chemicals that may affect our health. With this, there are now companies that create and produce organic skin care products. However again, this is just one part of nurturing and nourishing the skin. Our efforts to nurture it from the outside become incomplete if we don't eat the right and healthy foods.

In nourishing our skin through consumption of good food completes our goal of making our skin look healthy and youthful. That is why many of us include a lot of fruits and vegetables in our daily meals to ensure that we get all the vitamins, minerals and anti oxidants needed for our skin's health. However, as busy mothers or career women, we don't usually have the time to prepare healthy meals. That is why many of us are looking for easier and more convenient alternatives to ensure that we and our family enjoy palatable and at the same time guilt free meals. When it comes to skin care, juicing has become the craze today as it allows us to get almost all of the nutrients that we need in just one glass of fresh juice from different fruits and vegetables. This has been the talk for so many women. But is juicing really helpful in taking care of your skin? Or it only worsens the condition? The answer is it depends on your diet program and how you treat juicing. To clear these issues, we can consider the case of Hollywood celebrity Jennifer Aniston who treats juicing as part of her normal consumption of meals. This means that she does not undergo pure juicing diet or never resorted to juicing diet at all. She still eats the regular meals she follows everyday and drinks fresh juice as part of her daily consumption.

On the other hand, many food experts say that the juicing diet does more harm than good. According to Dr. Sam Bunting, a cosmetic dermatologist, your skin will dry up if you follow a juicing diet. This is because your skin does not get the essential fatty acids it needs. Furthermore, he said that if your skin is always prone to dryness you may experience development of patches of eczema. This is because the barrier function of the skin is compromised if it does not get the enough amounts of essential fatty acids.

Sticking to pure juicing diet also has long term effects that would horrify you. Juicing diet is low in calorie and this makes the insulin levels to spike and crash. Initially, this causes break outs. This insulin cycle alters the structures of elastin and collagen in the body over time. As a result, they become stiffer. This causes the skin to look prematurely old, which women never dream of. What we want is to maintain a youthful and glowing skin.

So, if you really want to get all the benefits of fresh juice from organic fruits and vegetables follow the recommendation of dietitian Natalie Jones. She said that it would be best if you have fresh juice as one of your five a day. She further said than consuming more than that won't do you any more good. It won't give you extra benefits but rather more harm.

Juicing for Healthy and Vibrant Hair

Aside from our skin, our hair is another part that we need to nurture and nourish. AS said it is our crowning glory and, thus, we have to ensure that it gets all the nutrients necessary for it to look shiny and silky. Today, there are also a lot of hair products that we patronize. Some of these are shampoo, hair conditioner, hot oil, hair dye, and others. Again, like commercial skin care products, these also have chemicals that may do harm to our hair later on in our life. To address this, many are now also resorting to organic hair products. However, these products are usually more expensive than the commercial ones. With this, juicing seems to be the most effective and yet more affordable alternative. But like juicing for skin care, it may also do you more harm than good if you don't do the right thing. What then is the right thing to do? How should we treat juicing in so far as nourishing the hair is concerned?

If you do away with your normal five a day and replace it with more fresh juice, you may suffer from hair loss later on. If you think you are getting all the nutrients from fresh juice you wouldn't know how to explain it. According to Philip Kingsley, a renowned trichologist, you may experience hair fall two to three months after you start your juicing diet. He said that he had seen women coming to him with unexplained hair loss. But after some discussions, it turned out that there were following an extreme juicing diet.

According to him, hair loss happens when the body stops producing hair. If the body does not get all the nutrients it needs, it powers down or stops the processes that it considers not essential to life. One is the production of hair. With extreme juicing, or pure juicing diet, you definitely don't get to have all the nutrient, vitamins and minerals that your body needs for it to perform all the functions and processes well. For sure, you would not want to lose hair and get bald. As women, we should know these as we may have a different or misleading presumption for our hair loss. One possible that we may think is cancer symptoms when it is only about the harms of extreme juicing diet.

Now that we know these things, we can make juice recipes that will nourish our hair but without compromising other nutrients that the body needs. For example, we can have fresh juice made out of fruits and vegetables that are good for the hair, and drink it as part of our morning or afternoon snack.

Juicing for Healthy Nails

Though the skin is biggest and most recognizable part of our body, the nails also reflect our health. We are not getting all the nutrients that our body needs if our nails look dull, brittle and has some white spots. This means that we are lacking certain vitamins and minerals. There are many ways by which this can be addressed. One way is through the use of nails products like nail polish. However, this is just like a band aid solution as it does not really address the nutrient deficiency of our body. One great way to have healthy nails is to adopt juicing. It is more practical than purchasing nail products. Your nails can look their best if you let them breathe. So, it can only breathe if you stop using nail polish. It should not be hard for you to let go of nail cosmetics a you can save money from it. Your nails will also look their best if you drink fresh juice using certain fruits and vegetables known to provide nourishment to your nails. Drinking fresh juice allows your nails to grow beautifully and stay strong.

To be effective in nourishing your nails, you have to consider nutrients and vitamins that are necessary in making your nails complete. This means that you are effective in the assimilation of all the nutrients from the juice you consume. So, you need to consider fruits and vegetables that are rich in Biotin, Zinc, Vitamin C and Omega 3 fatty acids. However, if you just eat these foods it would be a little harder for the nutrients to get into your bloodstream. But if you get these nutrients through juicing, it becomes easier for them to directly get into your bloodstream.

For your nails, you can use carrots, bananas, ginger, nuts, broccoli and leafy green varieties to create your juice. Combinations of these fruits and vegetables can give your skin the nutrients it needs such as Vitamin C and essential fatty acids. For example, if you want a juice high in Vitamin C, you can combine lemons, apples, ginger root and lime. If you want a juice rich in Omega 3 fatty acids, Biotin and Zinc, you can use pears, spinach and walnuts. Depending on what your nails need, there are specific fruits and vegetables that you have to combine. There are also juice recipes that you can follow if you want to achieve certain goals like longer and stronger nails. For this, you can use kale leaves without the stem, apricots with pits removed, mangoes, handfuls of blueberries, chia seeds, and green or red grapes.

Juicing for Beauty and Anti----Aging Purposes

There is no denying, fresh juice from fruits and vegetables can really make you beautiful and more youthful. With these, you might want to know what are some of the fruit and vegetables that you always have to keep in your refrigerator. Some of these are carrots, cucumbers and strawberries.

Carrots should always be present in your kitchen as it is rich in Vitamin C, which helps in promoting healthy eyesight. It also has antioxidants which help in boosting the immune system. This is essential especially nowadays that there are a lot of viruses and bacteria that may easily cause our sickness. Carrots taste really good when you combine them with apples. Cucumbers also contain Vitamin C. It has potassium and iron. It is highly recommended for women who want to flush out heavy toxins from their bodies through gentle detoxification. This is because the cucumber is a mild diuretic and is mostly made up of water. These promote frequent urination which is a way of flushing out toxins from your body.

Strawberries, unlike vegetables such as spinach, are more desirable. A strawberry is also high in Vitamin C, which helps in maintaining a strong immune system. It is also known to have antioxidants that fight free radicals. For people who suffer from arthritis, strawberries are good for them as these are anti inflammatory. Lastly, strawberries are essential in maintaining strong and healthy connective tissues such as bones and skins.

With the wonders of fresh juice from fruits and vegetables, women can now have a more affordable, healthier, safer and more enjoyable way of caring for their skin, hair and nails. They can now live without the commercially produced cosmetic products which have a lot of chemicals and preservatives. Juicing is definitely a lot better as it nourishes your skin, hair

and nails from the inside. If you are well fed with the nutrients you need, it will reflect on the outside. You don't have to use band aid solutions anymore. You just have to remember that you can optimize juicing to your advantage if you use organic produce and if you include juicing as one of your five a
day. You can even improve your youthful look by applying organic beauty products on
your skin, hair and nails.

7. Juicing for Vitality

Stress

The most common cause of sexual dysfunction is stress. The latter basically keeps your mind and body tired, unable to function at its most capable extent, turn your energy levels down, and leaves you out of time for love and other things aside from your career (or your household chores). This is why some people say that sex and satisfaction is just for men married men, that is. While women, who are tied to taking care of their children, or career women who are focused on excelling and succeeding among others, often lose their desire for orgasm and all the good things that come before that.

The human body has its limits and once these are reached, other tasks are not fulfilled. Stress and over fatigue comes from too much work whether at home or not. Women are generally turned on and become sexually excited through mental and emotional means. Unlike men who are visually aroused in general, women need some sort of sensual foreplay to get aroused. If they are mentally and emotionally stressed, the physical stage of getting excited for sex is blocked. Stressed women find it more difficult to reach orgasm when they are exhausted. This is because stress weakens the brains ability to send signals to the body, and therefore impairs our endocrine glands to do their work.

Aside from having the right juicing diet, you must learn to destress and unwind. Conscious efforts to reduce factors that add to your stress levels will definitely contribute to having more vitality in life. Make sure to have breaks every once in a while, go on vacations, listen to relaxing music, or simply take time to lay down in bed and have enough rest from your daily routine. There are a lot of stress reduction programs and techniques that you can use to make your juicing work at its fullest capacity.

Unhealthy Lifestyle

Having an unhealthy lifestyle does not only affect your overall well being. It largely affects your vitality and how good you do in bed. Do not wonder if you keep trying to get that groove back but are having a hard time getting full pleasure after having rounds of beer. Everyone, whether male or female, become less active in bed after getting some booze.

Alcohol naturally impairs our senses and thus affects our ability to participate in sexual activities and lowers down the production of testosterone, a hormone needed to boost your libido to its normal level. It is true that taking red wine regularly in limited and planned amounts is healthy for women who need to relax. However, taking more than two glasses will have negative effects on your sexual performance, and should be avoided if you want to have some romantic nights with your partner.

Likewise, the intake of too much caffeine (whether from coffee, tea, chocolate, etc.) interjects with the production of hormones, and in fact interferes with women's menstrual cycles. This means that your libido is also affected by excessive drinking of coffee. If you are addicted to any of these caffeine rich and addictive drinks, you might as well limit your intake. Otherwise, juicing might not just work for you.

While chocolates can act as aphrodisiacs for men, women who want to get some vitality up should avoid taking too much of these sweets.

Another factor that largely contributes to an unhealthy lifestyle that may affect your libido is smoking. Aside from the unwanted smell that it may cause your breath, smoking can be an overall killer for your love life. Because of the numerous toxins found in tobacco smoke, your body's oxygen will dramatically decrease and may cause blood vessel damage, and therefore decreases blood flow. Good blood circulation is vital in arousal, and contributes to the pleasure that you get from making love. So it is just right to say that anyone who needs some groovy nights should eliminate bad habits such as smoking, where lead, nicotine, cadmium, carbon monoxide, benzopyrene and a lot of other toxic chemicals take its toll through the most unwanted diseases such as cancer. Having illnesses such as cancer and losing your vitality would be the last thing you would want to happen to your busy life.

Aside from toxins you can get from smoking, people from all over the world today suffer from artificial food ingredients and chemicals that likewise inhibit good blood circulation, and lessen your energy for life's most exciting details. Preservatives, additives, artificial flavorings, coloring, and pesticides are big culprits for the human race's dwindling state of health. These chemicals bombard our bodies and take the place of the necessary nutrients that we need in order to perform well at work or in bed.

Not having enough sleep also brings your energy levels down, and obviously takes you out of the mood for love (or anything else other than sleep, that is!). It is vital to know that even if you have the most helpful juicing diet, the lack of sleep will still haunt you and keep you out of your groove.

Hormonal Imbalance and Changes

Hormonal changes and imbalances caused by stress, biological impairments, or natural life events such as menstrual cycles, postpartum phases, and menopause, similarly affect your libido. Hormonal imbalances often trigger physical discomfort, most commonly characterized by mood swings, insomnia, hot flashes, digestive problems, and weight gain. When a woman nears her menstrual period, or has just given birth or undergone abortion, hormonal levels change drastically. The physical byproducts directly affect her gusto for romance and lovemaking. Nonetheless, hormonal imbalances brought about by menstruation, postpartum phases, and abortion naturally settle down unless you are in need of some medical attention. Once your hormones get back to their normal levels, the physical challenges will also go away and leave you more comfortable doing anything and give you back your groove.

Libido is attributed to testosterone the life force hormone that gets us going on and on in bed. Having low testosterone levels is equivalent to low libido. The roots of low testosterone levels may be stress, or medical conditions that cause their ovaries to function abnormally.

Now that you know the reasons for having low sexual vitality, the next thing to do is to see if you are one of the majority of women who suffer from loss of sexual appetite. This is crucial information that will help you seek the best juicing recipes apt for your particular condition.

Are You Losing Your Vitality?

There is more to juicing than a fit and healthy body. With the correct combination of your most favorite vegetables, fruits, and herbs that make up perfect recipes, you can even revive your sexual vitality without having to take synthetic medicine. There are a few things you can check to see if you are indeed losing your vitality.

The first thing you should ask yourself is "Am I significantly, but unexplainably losing my appetite for sex?". To answer this question, you can take note of the frequency of your initiative or your partner's granted initiatives to have sex. Low libido is demonstrated by indifference, the inability to perk up for sex. Women are opposite to men as we grow older, our sex drive naturally stays longer because of increasing testosterone production. Males, as they get older, little by little lose their stride in bed because their production of testosterone decreases. This means that as you age, you must consider checking on your vitality, and see if it coincides with this fact. Lesser libido also means taking more time before reaching orgasm, or having less pleasurable orgasms than before. Yes, orgasms differ at one time or another. The intensity of that blissful moment where you feel all your muscles contracting can be discerned and that is a factor you must consider. You may still be having sex in as frequent as you used to do, but the climax and the pleasure is another thing to look after. Sex is not just a routine it is humans greatest gift of expression and should therefore serve its purpose: to make you feel love and loved in return. Sex without orgasm is just like doing your household chores or work assignments it will only leave you exhausted and unfulfilled at the end of the day. So if you are often faced with exhaustion after having sex, you might be losing your groove unconsciously.

A lot of women suffer from the above mentioned factors due to loss of vaginal lubrication. The latter likewise shows they need more groove back.

If you are experiencing any of these, there is indeed a great need for you to focus on the right juicing recipes that will help you get your vitality return to its normal phase.

Juicing for Vitality

A lot of women, as they age, have less and less sex due to many reasons. Some women do not have sex at all. And what's the reason behind this? Generally, they lose their interest in lovemaking or they simply do not make time for it. Women who are at their 40's and beyond go through menopause, which some consider the end of sexual pleasure. However, contrary to this common misconception, menopause is actually another exciting stage in a woman's life wherein having sex no longer leaves you worried of getting an unplanned pregnancy. Then again, the hormonal imbalance it causes makes it a bit hard for women to enjoy this supposedly stimulating stage.

There are a lot of juicing recipes and suggested ingredients that are particularly advised for women who suffer from hormonal imbalance and loss of sexual vitality thereafter. A combination of beet, carrot, and ginger, with a hint of grape juice, helps bring back your hormonal levels to normal.

Squash, when juiced, adds to your body's production of the right hormones that will take your sexual desires up. Add a bit of cinnamon regularly to your daily dose of juice and you can expect to be ready for sex anytime. There is a huge difference between aphrodisiacs and juicing for sexual vitality. The latter revives your energy and gives you most oomph in bed. Aphrodisiacs, on the other hand, simply makes you go hot and do not necessarily keep you in the groove. It is just to say that they will not make your orgasms more intense and the whole sexual experience more pleasurable.

Seeds and nuts, like sesame, sunflower, pumpkin seeds, chia, and hemp are best juiced with fruits. Beans and grains are likewise best for those who want to add vitality to their lives. Adding a bit of garlic, ginger, and cardamom gives a little flavor to your recipe, and likewise warms up your body as you would need it for some hot and romantic nights.

To help your blood circulate, make your body ready for complete and necessary arousal for a good sexual intercourse, turmeric, cayenne, and lemon will be the perfect addition to your juicing recipe. Regular intake of these healthy ingredients will help your blood circulate throughout your body, including your vagina and everything that surrounds it. Opposite to what we commonly believe, males are not alone in the need for excellent blood circulation to pump up their penis during lovemaking.

It also helps to include acai, berried, cruciferous vegetables, and mangosteen to your daily dose of healthy juicing recipes to promote a healthy liver. In return, your liver does its job in your body's blood circulation.

Here is an example of a juicing recipe for women in search of good vitality:

Prepare 4 carrots. Make sure to leave it half peeled as the skin is the healthiest part of this root. Add 2 stalks of celery.

Celeries are rich in androsterone, a hormone that helps stimulates your sex drive. Add in 3 kale leaves and half a cucumber that will increase your libido and stamina. Use one knuckle of ginger to remove toxins in your blood and promote good blood circulation.

Another juicing recipe that will help bring your groove back:

Ingredients:

1.   1 large bulb of fennel (make sure to remove fronds and trim it)
2.   2" ginger knob
3.   3 ripe pears (best to choose organic ones to avoid unwanted chemicals and toxins)
4.   1 large bunch of watercress
5.   1 lemon

Cut the fennel bulb and pears into four parts. Peel and remove the pith from the lemon. Slice it in half. Place everything inside a juicer. Drink immediately to avoid separation of parts.

Juicing recipes are not hard to prepare. They involve a bit of slicing, paring, and peeling, and all you have to do is use a juicer to create than wonderful drink that will bring you vitality.

Here are other juicing recipe suggestions for a more active sex life:

Combine 4 kale leaves, half a cup of mango, 5 romaine leaves, half a cup of pineapple, half a cup of parsley sprigs, and half an inch slice of ginger. This powerful combination gives you a green smoothie that will bring your energy in bed back in no time. It is overall detoxifying, and helps boost blood circulation for an ultimate climax.

You can also try juicing 1 apple, half a cup of parsley or spinach, 4 unpeeled carrots, and 1 pared kiwi. This recipe is an energizer that will give you more drive as you feel your youthfulness once again.

A glass of pomegranate juice each day also brings your testosterone levels up, and therefore makes you yearn for sex.

The key to making an effective and enjoyable vitality juice that will bring your groove back is to know the basic ingredients (vegetables, fruits, nuts, roots, and the like) that basically promote good blood circulation, relaxation, more energy, better health and mood.

On the other hand, your efforts in juicing for vitality may reach its full potential in bringing back your sex appetite if you are not wary of the kind of food that you eat. As said in the previous chapters, it is crucial to choose your food if you are serious in practicing a healthy lifestyle, not to mention trying to regain your sexual vitality.

The following foods are a no no for women who want to real and effective juicing for a more healthy and satisfying sex life:

1.   Fried food. Trans fats that come from fried food lower libido levels by clogging your blood vessels and veins and therefore giving your blood a hard time to circulate all throughout your body. The effect? Your senses do not get as sensitive as they should, your sexual organs have lower reaction capabilities to romance stimulus, and all in all you lose your passion for sex and orgasm.

If you prefer to somehow eat your regular meals other than juicing, make sure to use healthy and proper cooking procedures that do not use oil, chemicals, or other toxins that will ruin your juicing diet. Try steaming or boiling your food to avoid unwanted fats.

2.   Soy products. Soy products, although were believed to be of good benefit to people's health, have been found to promote higher levels of estrogen. In various studies done all

over the world, people have proven that soy is one of the culprits for hormonal imbalance and takes away women's sex drive. A little amount should be okay, but daily big doses will mean a lot of negative effects on your body, including but not limited to sexual impotence and loss of interest.

3.   High fat dairy. This can be found in cheese, ice cream, and milkshake which can aggravate pre menstrual cycle syndromes and dysmenorrhea. Worst, high dairy fat can lower down your libido as well.

4.   Combination of flour and sugar. Yes, you read that right. Anything that is made out of combined flour and sugar is a no no. It combats our genuine objective to increase our vitality and get our groove back. Cupcakes, cakes, cookies, macaroons, muffins, brownies, and the like amplifies our glucose levels, and in turn causes hormonal imbalance and decreases our appetite for sex and romance.

Make sure to balance your diet and stick with those that can help boost your vitality. Juicing is an effective way to bring your groove back, but without the proper diet and exercise, you cannot expect to get the best results. Similarly, it is crucial to have a balanced and healthy lifestyle that enables your body to recuperate from all the hassles of being a superwoman, and gives you the space and time to care for yourself. Remember, reviving your appetite and energy for sex is affected by physical, mental, and emotional conditions.

Once you have managed to renew your lifestyle to a healthier one, change your diet to fit your juicing recipes, and maintained your intake of vitality juices, your love life will give you the best and most romantic love making experience—something you can call a
reward for living such a healthy life.

8. Improving Overall Health

The biggest question to most people who are new to juicing: What exact difference does it have compared to eating fruits and vegetables as a whole?

Vegetarians and vegans basically stick with the same ingredients as what juicing uses. Overall, eating vegetables and fruits as your main diet, combined with good sources of protein such as beans, nuts, and seeds, gives your body a complete set of nutrients that is needed for it to function well. To start giving you an idea of the health benefits of juicing, here is a detailed elucidation of what vegetables and fruits fundamentally provide our bodies.

Knowing the health benefits: Introduction to vitamins and minerals from veggies and fruits

Vitamin A is essential in the reproduction of cells, and helps build strong immunity against diseases. Some hormones are produced sufficiently with the support of this nutrient. It also promotes good eyesight, bone and teeth development, and contributes to how your hair and skin shines and glows. Vitamin A is found in vegetables like Bok Choy, Amaranth Leaves, Butternut, Broccoli, Chinese Broccoli, Squash, Carrots, Leeks, Kale, spinach, pumpkin, sweet potato, and cabbage. Fruits such as grapefruit, papaya, mango, cantaloupes, guava, watermelon, and tomatoes are a good source of Vitamin A. Vitamin B1, also called thiamine, boosts your energy and therefore makes you go through your day despite your hectic schedule. It is fundamental in converting carbohydrates into useful energy. Most importantly, it promotes full function for the nervous system, the heart, and muscles. Thiamine deficiency leads to fatigue and weakness. This powerful vitamin can be found in vegetables such as spirulina, asparagus, butternut, corn, lima beans, peas, parsnips, sweet potato, Brussels sprouts, French beans, and okra. Fruits rich in thiamine are boysenberries, avocado, dates, guava, breadfruit, grapes, mango, loganberries, cherimoya, pineapple, watermelon, pomegranate, and grapefruit.

Riboflavin, otherwise known as vitamin B2, is an essential factor for normal body growth. It is likewise important in reproducing red cells. Like thiamine, it helps release energy from carbohydrates. Vegetables rich in riboflavin are artichoke, amaranth leaves, Brussels sprouts, asparagus, lima beans, mushrooms, bok choy, chineses broccoli, peas, sweet potato, peas, and swiss chard. Fruits that give you riboflavin are banana, avocado, dates, passion fruit, cherimoya, grapes, pomegranate, lychee, mulberries, prickly pear, and mangoes.

Vitamin B3 is another essential vitamin that the body gets from different foods. It is also called niacin, and it promotes a healthy digestive system. It also helps the skin and nerves to function. Like the previous two, niacin assists in converting carbohydrates to useful energy. Parsnips, spirulina, okra, artichoke, butternut, corn, squash, and peas are just a few of the many vegetables that provide us with this vitamin. Fruits such as boysenberries, dates, avocado, passion fruit, nectarine, peaches, and guava are among those which contain niacin.

Pantothenic acid or vitamin B5 helps produce hormones and good cholesterol which are vital in maintaining a healthy body. It is found in broccoli, squash, butternut, okra, mushrooms, corn, French beans, among others. Black currants, avocado, gooseberries, dates, cherimoya, raspberries, watermelon, starfruit, grapefruits, and breadfruit are also good sources of vitamin B5.

The same vegetables are also rich in vitamin B6, which contributes in creating antibodies for your immune system. Also called pyridoxine, this vitamin has a big role in processing protein intake. For people who have big intakes of protein, bigger amounts of pyridoxine is likewise needed. Otherwise, the person will suffer from convulsions, dizziness, confusion, and nausea.

Vitamin B9, which is found in most fruits and vegetables mentioned above, is essential in producing red blood cells and the nervous system. Women who plan to become pregnant should have sufficient intake of vitamin B9, which comes in the form of folate and folic acid.

Vitamin C is another essential vitamin that the body needs in order to have full function. It acts as an antioxidant that protects human cells from the bad effects of free radicals. It is also a good antiviral agent that blocks viral diseases. Amaranth leaves, broccoli, bok choy, butternut, squash, kale, green pepper, and swiss chard are vegetables with vitamin C. Fruits rich in vitamin C are strawberries, pineapples, mulberries, black currants, grapefruits, breadfruits, lychee, oranges, mangoes, kiwi, papaya, and passion fruit.

Vitamin E is another antioxidant that protects our bodies from oxidation damages. It also plays a significant role in the creation of red blood cells. It is vital and indispensable in putting vitamin K into use. Vitamin E is used by women to reduce scars and wrinkles, as it can heal broken skin tissues. This particular vitamin is found in a lot of fruits (i.e. blackberries, guava, avocado, black currants, breadfruit, blueberries, cranberries, boysenberries, loganberries, kiwi, papaya, mango, nectarine, mulberries, peaches, pomegranate, peach, and raspberries.

Most of the above mentioned vegetables and fruits likewise contain vitamin K, which has an important part in blood clotting. This vitamin is essential in regulating calcium levels in the blood, and activates proteins that add to maintaining healthy bones. Chinese pears, plums, tomatoes, alfalfa sprouts, cauliflower, celery, cucumber, and rapini are a few more vegetables that provide vitamin K to our bodies.

Vitamin D maintains our calcium and phosphorus levels in the blood. It helps the body absorb calcium and magnesium, and therefore promotes good and healthy bone and teeth development. Mushrooms are the only vegetables (or non meat product, rather) that contains vitamin D.

On the down side, Vitamin B12, which plays an important role in your body's metabolism, cannot be found in vegetables and fruits. Fish, meat, poultry, and dairy products are the only food that act as sources of vitamin B12.

Vegetables and fruits are also rich in essential minerals that the body needs. We have already mentioned how calcium and magnesium play and important role in bone development. Calcium likewise lessens insomnia and promotes the correct contraction of muscles, clotting of blood, and efficient functioning of the nerves. Copper helps the body absorb and use iron, and thus contributes to the formation of red blood cells. Consequently, it promotes good supply of oxygen to the body, which in turn allows for better nutrient absorption.

Iron, which comes from most fruits, is especially found in raisins. Manganese, Phosphorus, Potassium, Selenium, Sodium, and Zinc are other minerals found in most vegetables.

Now that you are familiar with all the vitamins and minerals that can be found in vegetables and fruits, let us answer the first question that was asked earlier in this chapter. What exact difference does it have compared to eating fruits and vegetables as a whole?

Benefits of Juicing

Juicing, unlike eating your vegetables and fruits in whole, makes it easier for the body to absorb all the nutrients in them. A lot of people suffer from digestive problems, and juicing somehow digest the food for them. Instead of worrying what type of food will be easier for them to digest, they will now have to pay attention to the vitamins and minerals that they need in order to maintain a healthy diet.

Today's fast food filled world suggest more meat and artificial diets rather than eating healthy, fresh, and chemical free. Children are brought up at McDonald's, literally spend their birthdays there, and are trained to love unhealthy foods over healthy vegetables. This makes it very difficult for them to eat vegetables despite the need for it. If you are one of those who were overshadowed by the McDonald dream, juicing can be a huge help for you to start taking more veggies without the torment. One glass of vegetable juice may be sufficient to supply your body with enough vitamins and minerals that you need—given that you are able to combine the right ingredients as you add juicing to your diet.

Juicing is a fun way to enhance your diet and give your body an overall boost from stress and illnesses. You can add different flavors to your not so loved vegetables to make them taste more palatable, or do an experiment on your favorite fruits.

Juicing Against Cancer

Cancer is one of the greatest fears of Americans when it comes to their health. It is one of the most common causes of death, and is still rising at present. There are many things that contribute to why cases of cancer are increasing. Generally, cancer is caused by different factors including genetics, chemicals from smoking tobacco, unhealthy diet and abnormal physical activities, overexposure to the sun's UV rays, exposure to radiation, and other carcinogens.

Some families genetically pass on cancer from one generation to another. However, this does not necessarily mean that all families with cancer patients from different generations have hereditary cancer. Different generations in a family with multiple cancer patients often inherit other types of disease that increase the risk of cancer. In reality, cancer itself cannot be inherited. People inherit abnormal genes that may lead to certain types of cancer. This constitutes only 5-10% of all cancers.

This being said, we can easily state that even 'inherited' cancer can be prevented by following a healthy diet and lifestyle. This is contrary to popular belief that 'inherited' cancer is inevitable.

Cigarette smoking is identified as the "major single cause of cancer mortality [death] in the United States", according to the 1982 report from the United States Surgeon General. 16.5% of adult women smoke cigarettes—the same culprit for 30% of all deaths caused by cancer. 87% of the deaths among lung cancer patients is caused by smoking. Second hand smoke is also a cause of cancer. Although there is still a need for further studies and evidences, second hand smoke has been seen to cause breast cancer among women.

Likewise, smoking is strongly attributed to lung cancer, oral cavity cancers, larynx cancer, esophagus and pharynx cancers, stomach, pancreas, cervix, kidney, bladder, ovarian, colorectum cancers, and acute myeloid leukemia.

The most common type of cancer in women in the US is breast cancer. However, the most common cause of cancer death among women is still lung cancer. Causes of breast cancer vary as well—from aging, genetics, history of breast cancer, breast lumps, exposure to estrogen, obesity, exposure to radiation and carcinogens, and implants. To prevent breast cancer, a good and healthy lifestyle should be developed. It has also been learned that breast cancer survivors are more likely to have diabetes.

Fortunately, there are many vegetables and fruits that contain nutrients that act as antioxidants and prevent cancer. Carrot juice helps in detoxifying the body, particularly the liver, and helps flush out excess fat and unwanted chemicals (those that you get from eating genetically modified products, artificial flavorings and additives). As your liver functions to its full capacity, your fats are easily burned and thus keeps you away from being overweight. Prevention of the latter contributes in preventing different types of cancer. Beets add more detoxifying agents to your body and further pushes toxic chemicals out of your body. Drinking beet juice in large amounts is known to terminate cancers and tumors in the body.

Cabbage, which is rich in vitamins and minerals, is also a good choice to combine with carrot juice. As long as it is pesticide free, cabbages consumed regularly help in preventing cancer just as studies show.

Green leafy vegetables are high sources of antioxidants, and promote the formation of red blood cells. Most green and leafy vegetables contain almost all essential vitamins and minerals, so juicing them will be perfect for those who want to make sure their bodies are fully maintained.

Juicing Against Diabetes

Diabetes is an illness that is demonstrated by a complex of different diseases like hyperglycemia. Diabetes happens when your body does not produce enough insulin that will help your body absorb and transform glucose into energy. Insulin comes from the pancreas.

There are two types of diabetes—type 1 and type 2 diabetes. Type 1 diabetes is caused by the inability of the pancreas to produce insulin because its beta cells are destructed by the body's immune system. This happens when there is an autoimmune deficiency. Although type 1 diabetes is not caused by a virus, experts suggest they are closely link to each other. On the other hand, type 2 diabetes is the most common type of diabetes among US and non----US citizens. It is caused by multiple factors, which is worsened by the body's inability to efficiently make use of insulin. The most overpowering factor is having a family history of this kind of illness. Obesity, an inactive lifestyle, aging, and unhealthy diet contribute to the risk of having type 2 diabetes. Other illnesses such as pancreatitis or pancreatectomy, glucagonoma, polycystic ovary syndrome, and steroid induced diabetes also potential causes of type 2 diabetes.

In the US, more than 12.6 million women aged 20 years and beyond suffer from diabetes. 68% of diabetics (who are 65 years old and above) have heart disease. 67% of people with diabetes who are 20 years old and above have high blood pressure. As much as 70% of diabetics suffer from different forms of nervous system injury. In 2007, diabetes was found to have played a role in the death of more than 231,000 deaths. Good thing there is a wide array of juicing recipes especially prepared for diabetics. Since diabetes is a complex group of diseases characterized with insufficient production of insulin or ineffective use of insulin (or both) causing hyperglycemia, there are a lot of vegetables and juices you can use to prevent risk factors from developing. A lot of vegetables and fruits are beneficial to diabetics as they help the body respond to insulin better, and give type 2 diabetics an easier way to trim down their bodies.

The basics of juicing for diabetics should begin with knowing what you need to avoid: glucose, sucrose, and fructose. Glucose is basically the type of sugar that comes from carbohydrates when broken down by the human body. Fructose is naturally found in fruits. Glucose and fructose is sucrose when combined.

To avoid sucrose, it is wiser for diabetics to stick with a vegetable juicing diet. However, one of the disadvantages of juicing is that it does not give as much fiber as eating whole vegetables do. Then again, by choosing the right vegetables that do not contain much carbohydrates, you will be able to stay away from complications and take advantage of the positive effects of juicing. Other people choose not to peel their vegetables so they can still get enough fiber that is very effective in regulating blood sugar.

Juicing recipes for diabetics are made up of non----starchy veggies which have small amounts of carbohydrates and contain a low glycemic index. However, studies show that processing food increases its glycemic index. This means that vegetable juice will probably contain a higher glycemic index compared to vegetables when eaten as a whole.

Asparagus is known to help keep sugar levels down. The intake of tomatoes, cucumber, Brussels sprouts, and cucumber contributes to the management of diabetes. Vegetables rich in manganese are good in keeping insulin resistance down. Vitamin C is an effective tool to prevent diabetes, and can be found in broccoli.

Cinnamon is likewise known to help in lowering resistance to insulin, and therefore promotes better insulin sensitivity. Adding cinnamon to your vegetable juice does not only have the positive effects to your body, but is easy to find, and incorporate to recipes, and adds a twist to boring juices.

Green leafy vegetables like spinach, kale, and collards are among the most nutritious and diabetic friendly foods that you can use in your juicing recipe against diabetes. A combination of carrots, cucumber, spinach, celery, and a small slice of green apple works for those who need some nutrient boost without taking too much glucose and fructose.
Tomatoes can be combined with green pepper, ginger, celery, and garlic. You can also try to juice romaine lettuce with celery and tomatoes. Asparagus, carrots, and zucchini are also a perfect match to tomato juice.

Juicing Against Digestive Problems

Digestive problems are very common in Americans, which can be attributed to the growing unhealthy lifestyle in the country. There are many forms of digestive problems, ranging from short lived reflux, to peptic ulcers, gallstones, chronic constipation, abdominal wall hernia, diverticular disease, gastrointestinal infections, inflammatory bowel disease, irritable bowel syndrome, ulcerative colitis, liver disease, peptic ulcer disease, pancreatitis, viral hepatitis, and hemorrhoids.

In the US, 60 to 70 million people have some type of digestive problem. The most common digestive disorder for women in the US is esophageal reflux, which is felt by 21.1% of the country's female population. Abdominal hernia comes next, followed by irritable bowel syndrome, constipation, and gallstones.

It is imperative for busy women to check on their digestive health and know what their lifestyle and eating habits are causing their digestive system. The first signs of having a problem is having regular heartburn. Bloating or flatulence due to gas is another symptom to look out for. It may sound a bit gross, but you also need to check on your stool to know whether you are up for a digestive problem or not. If you see blood, undigested food, or oil, then you might want to take note and ask for some professional advice. Diarrhea and constipation, as well as stomach pain when eating or defecation, vomiting, and belching are all symptoms of having some kind of digestive problem.

There are many causes for digestive issues, including health problems that contribute to how our digestive system reacts or functions. Food allergies, the body's inability to absorb nutrients properly, lactose intolerance, infections and issues in your immune system, intestinal wall deterioration, and other allergies are risk factors.

If you have digestive issues, juicing is the most wonderful thing that has been invented for you. Because you have problems digesting your food effectively, juicing makes it possible for you to take in essential nutrients without having to worry about indigestion. The digestion is actually done for you before you drink the juice. For a more effective juicing that will promote good digestion, you must include the pulp to your juice because it contains the needed fiber for your intestines and stomach. Fiber helps cleanse your digestive system and thus prevents problems in the future.

Vegetable juice is best for those who have digestive issues or are conscious of their digestive health since fruit juice contains a lot of fructose. Starchy vegetables also contain higher levels of sugar than green, leafy or non starchy veggies. But for those who love fruits, a good juicing recipe for digestion is a combination of 4 kiwifruit, ¼ lime, 2 medium sized apples, 1 pineapple, ¼ lemon with rind, and 2 peeled oranges juiced together. This is best served cold as a refreshing juice drink.

For whatever particular purpose you have when juicing, always base your recipes on the basics of your objective (Are you juicing to prevent cancer? What causes cancer, then? What things should you avoid? What type of vitamins and minerals help in preventing cancer?) And how it can be achieved (Where can these powerful vitamins and minerals be found?). Effective juicing can be done through correct knowledge and information, as well as continuous and regular intake of the right vegetable and fruit juices combined with proper meals and diet. By doing so, you can be sure that your body is well nourished, armed with strong immune system, and functions well to eliminate all the bad elements that you intake in all sorts of activities.

Women should particularly be aware of what juicing can do to their bodies once it is done correctly. So before you begin juicing, make sure you are well familiar with yourself first— know your body, your lifestyle, your mood and disposition, and your whole personality so that you can practice the right juicing habits. Remember, juicing must not make you feel unsatisfied. Rather, it should make you feel powerful, healthy, and contented. So if you are feeling a bit (or totally) deprived when you start juicing, you may want to start over and begin with the first steps to make sure you are doing it right. Otherwise, it may not do you any good as you expect.

9. Food Combinations

We have already discussed how we can experiment on our favorite vegetables and
fruits when juicing, and have constantly brought up the need to properly exercise juicing with the right diet—that which involves real, solid food. Juicing alone does not often causes unlikely effects such as that which were mentioned in the previous chapters. So keep in mind that unless you are doing it as a temporary and weight loss program, juicing without eating proper meals will bring you problems instead of solutions.

There is a proper combination of foods that will not make you suffer from indigestion or some other kind of digestion problem. Between vegetables and fruits or both, you must know what to and what not to combine. Between juicing and proper meals, you must be able to combine the right stuff to avoid high cholesterol, malnutrition, clogged arteries, gallstones, and other disorders such as food allergies and diarrhea, bloating, heartburn, weight gain, constipation, leaky gut syndrome, and many more.

The combination of acid and alkali (or starchy foods and protein rich foods), for example, is a bad food combination that will surely make you feel uncomfortable if not fully unable to function well.

Proper food combining allows for easy and ideal digestion, which in turn keeps you away from undigested food inside your stomach. Indigestion or the inability to digest your food properly will leave toxic waste inside your body, and results in nausea, stomach pain, and bloating. You would not want this to happen as you attend that special event in your best evening gown, so keep an eye on the food that you eat!

The usual American meal made of steak, potatoes, soda, and bread is a suicide when it comes to proper food combining.

As you get to your favorite restaurant, you start off with a cold soda which basically holds up your stomach's act of digesting whatever you are about to take. As you eat your bread, your digestive system focuses on it and forgets about your steak and potato as you eat them next. In a standstill, your stomach will then make you feel so full, bloated, and gassy.

Now, don't go believing that combining meat with fiber (fruits and vegetables) is always the right way to food combining. Eating fruits after a meal can also cause gas and bloating, contrary to what we commonly think. People think that eating a fruit or fruits after a heavy meal helps their bodies digest the heavy part. However, the contrary happens because fruits have fructose which is easy to process without the need for digestion. On the other hand, carbohydrates or protein need much more time to get digested and processed, and affects the fruit that you eat after your meal. Instead of being expelled sooner, the fruit will stay in your stomach for a longer period of time and will ferment. This is why you will get gas by doing this wrong habit.

Another bad habit wrongfully done in most cultures is the combination of protein rich ingredients or food such as with cheese and egg omelets. Combining starchy foods with protein such as in lasagna or sandwiches is another common mistake done in western or European culture. The combination of tomato sauce and cheese in pasta, pizza, or other Mexican dishes is a no no if you want optimum digestion. Juice, which is acidic, and milk or other forms of dairy are two incompatible ingredients that can diminish your ability to digest, and has the ability to cause allergies, sinusitis, colds, and cough. It is also a known cause of the production of toxins inside the body, so make sure you avoid yogurt with fruits, or oatmeal with milk and juice. Mixing melon fruit with milk is also not a good idea.

Good and Bad Food Combinations

"So what options do I have?" Surely, this is a question that is boggling your mind right now. All the food combinations that you believed were alright since they tasted like heaven are actually creating hell inside your digestive system.

Do not worry, as there are still a lot of choices left even if you start taking out these unhealthy food combinations on your daily recipes. There is still even a lot more options even as you introduce juicing to your body, and combine it with proper meals.

Food combining allows you to get all the important nutrients that you need. If you stick with one particular type of food, you may develop deficiency of other nutrients that are not present in your chosen food. A number of vegetables have most vitamins and minerals in them, but if you are seeking for a particular effect of juicing, not all vegetables may give the most positive results. Whether you are into juicing fruits or vegetables, there is a good combination that will help you get your ultimate objective. Unlike what most people think, mixing just any type of fruits together does not instantly make a healthy juice drink. You may be thinking that you are on a fruit diet but behind everything, you can be causing damage to your digestive system.

The basic rule when combining fruits is to avoid mixing acid fruits and sweet fruits together. Acid fruits take up to 2 hours to digest. Examples of these fruits are cranberries, grapefruits, sour apples, sour peaches, sour plums, loganberry, pomegranate, tomatoes, lime, current, orange, lemon, tangerine, pineapple, tangelo, and strawberries. Sweet fruits include bananas, mangoes, dates, raisin, fig, all dried fruits, papaya, persimmon, prunes, and sapote.

It is okay to combine acid fruits or sweet fruits with sub acid fruits like apricots, boysenberries, apples, blackberries, blueberries, cherimoyas, cherries, grapes, elderberries, huckleberries, fresh figs, guavas, kiwis, nectarines, mulberries, peaches, plums, passion fruits, pears, quince, prickly pear, and raspberries.

All kinds of melons (like Casaba, Cantaloupe, Banana melon, Christmas melon,
Crenshaw melon, Persian melon, Honeydew melon, Watermelon, Nutmeg melon, and
Muskmelon) are best eaten alone. They usually take at most two hours to digest.

Although fruits are commonly added to make our meals taste more enjoyable, they are best eaten on their own. Experts say that if you want to have regular snack, you can eat fruits on an empty stomach since they are easy to digest and doing so will prevent difficulties in digesting food.

Vegetables are classified into two categories: starchy and non starchy veggies. Low and non starchy vegetables are okay to combine with protein starch that comes from beans, soy beans, peas, and navy beans. You can also mix non starchy vegetables with protein fat from dairy products, avocado, nuts and seeds, olives, and butter, cream, and oils. Protein starch and fat take as much as 12 hours to digest, just like meat and poultry.
This is why when you eat a whole steak on your date, you will feel somewhat full until the next morning (or maybe until lunch!) since that piece of meat is giving your stomach a hard time doing its job.

Non starchy vegetables are green, leafy ones, and bamboo shoots, bell pepper, cabbage, cauliflower, broccoli, eggplant, mung bean sprouts, mushrooms, okra, radish, turnip, sea vegetables, artichokes, alfalfa sprouts, beets, Brussels sprouts, asparagus, chard, carrots, leeks, garlic, scallions and many more.

Starchy vegetables take up to five hours before they get digested, just like non starchy vegetables. They are fine when combined with the latter, since they practically take the same amount of time to digest. Anything that has a lot of carbohydrates, potatoes, squash, chestnuts, pumpkin, corn, grains, and Jerusalem artichoke are examples of starchy vegetables that you should not combine with meat and poultry, as well as protein rich dairy and even fruits. After all, fruit and vegetable intermixing should be avoided unless you are prepared for some gaseous experience!

Take a look at how you usually eat—what type of food you prepare for breakfast, lunch, dinner, and in between snacks. You will realize that without knowing it, you have been causing problems for your digestive system.

The typical idea of a "healthy meal" for an American is balancing the go, grow, and glow foods (carbohydrates, protein, and vegetables or fruits). This is seen is such a way that people just try to look for options when preparing their meals, and not scrutinize them effectively. For so long, even during our younger years, health conscious people who do not get proper education about food combining take so much time and effort in choosing their foods and preparing their meals, but people often eat oatmeal with milk and banana during breakfast, and they think they have fed themselves with a healthy combination of starch, fruits, and dairy. Quite oppositely, milk and banana combinations are considered toxic producing food combinations and slows down the body and mind's reaction. It is very difficult to digest milk and bananas altogether, so make sure that if you use this combination, choose to very ripe banana and add some nutmeg and/or cardamom to support digestion. Meanwhile, it is better to eat the oatmeal with milk and banana separately to avoid this problem. As fruits are best taken with an empty stomach, you can eat the banana ahead of time, and wait 30 minutes before eating your oatmeal.

If you are to practice juicing with regular meals, the correct combination of your daily juicing recipe and regular meals should be based on the right food combination we have discussed earlier.

If you are pregnant, or planning to get pregnant, juicing can cause you harm if you do not combine it with the right food match, or you are unable to balance your intake of the different types of fruits and vegetables. It is vital to ensure that you get complete nutrition for your health and your baby's. Therefore, your juicing and overall diet should be balanced, well combined, and planned based on pregnancy's necessities. You need additional folate or folic acid, iodine, iron, calcium, zinc, manganese, vitamin D, vitamin C, vitamin A in varying amounts. You must talk to your ob-gyne regarding the needed nutrients that you must consider as you plan for your meals.

Women who are always on the go should also be conscious about the kind of food that they eat. While they should have more carbohydrate or starch intake, it should be clear that eating pure carbs or starchy vegetables is going to be an unbalanced diet.

Eating chicken or fish with rice or any other food rich in carbohydrates is also unbeneficial to your health. Aside from giving you a lot of reasons to gain weight and lose control of your figure, this weight adding combination is a wrong choice that may leave you feeling bloated. Worse, you can have indigestion and get other digestive issues.

Bacon and eggs for breakfast represents the biggest killer in preserving a healthy diet. Bacon, aside from being a protein starch and protein fat rich food, has plenty of preservatives, and salt. When fried, it accrues more fats through the cooking oil. If you plan to waste your efforts in juicing to lose weight and return to your healthy self, then fried bacon and eggs will serve you the best results.

Pancakes are also commonly served with bananas or other sweet fruits for breakfast. Skip this as well. Both are high in sugar, and take different amounts of time for digestion, which makes them unhealthy for the busy career woman.

Peanut butter and jelly sandwich for your kids is also not a good idea, although a lot of parents prepare this for their children. Egg and toast, turkey sandwich, bagel and cream cheese are just a few more of the bad food pairings that play a huge role in the deterioration of your health. They are also part of the big syndicate that robs your body of the essential nutrients and cause the increase in toxins and thus lead you towards deadly medical conditions such as cancer, diabetes, and the like.

Now, you might be thinking that you have violated proper food combining all your life. Well, that is no longer surprising since most Americans practice such unhealthy lifestyles that circle on fast food chains and steak houses as they do not have enough time to cook and shop ingredients for themselves. Full time moms may have more chances of changing their family's health through implementing good food combinations. Career women and those who focus on their businesses are in great need of a diet reform—a change in their habits that will start with proper education on how and why food combining is done. Always keep in mind that in practicing good food combination, it is imperative to take away bad and unhealthy habits that will keep you from its potential benefits. Food combining and juicing are just two of the things you can do to help keep your body healthy. They, alone, are not enough to keep you healthy. You cannot expect to live long through proper food matching and regular juicing if you smoke cigarettes or drink excessive alcohol. The thing is, you just can't be healthy and live an unhealthy lifestyle at the same time.

Food combining is a good step towards a brighter and happier future. It enables you to build and maintain your body consciously. On the other hand, bad eating habits contravene the advantages and positive effects of proper food combining. There are a lot of these bad habits, but here are some to name a few:

Overindulging in fatty and starchy foods makes it hard for your body to produce enough juices needed to digest the amount of food you have taken. Limit your intake of fatty food and starchy fruits and vegetables, as well as carbohydrate rich grains and products. Do not take them together.

Drinking more than a small number of sips as you eat your meals interferes with your digestive system's enzyme secretion. It dilutes the enzymes that are responsible for the efficient digestion of your meal.

Stress eating, eating when you are tired, eating even when you are not hungry, and forcing yourself to eat foods that you really do not like also stops your body from benefiting well from food combining and juicing.

Eating before you are ready (or your stomach is ready) is another bad habit that counters your efforts in food combining and/or juicing. You can say that you are not yet ready for another meal if you are familiar with the length of time needed to digest all types of food. If you ate steak during your previous meal, make sure your stomach has completely digested (or at least close to it) the meat before eating another piece of meat. If you ate sweet or acidic fruits right after you ate your steak, you are probably suffering from fermenting debris in your stomach and therefore must not force yourself to eat.

Not chewing your food properly, or simply eating too quickly are both included in the list of bad habits which may interfere with your healthy routine.

Sleeping right after eating, as well as vigorously exercising will keep you away from your objectives as to why you are presently into juicing and food combining. The intake of too much seasonings and toxic irritants like onions, pepper, vinegar, and bitter herbs destroys your stomach's natural pH. Taking medicine is also a factor.

There are many things that food combining can bring and supplement juicing, but it is undeniably true that some dietitians and writers say that there is no need for food combining. Their reason boils down to one thing: they say that the human stomach was designed to digest about anything regardless of combination.

Still, we believe that humans have long spoken about their bodies based on real life experiences. Our bodies are not perfect, and they do not function the same. Depending on our particular health conditions, our stomachs work in different efficiency levels. Some stomachs are more sensitive and cannot tolerate too much protein, while some are able to digest them.

Food combining is a customizable program that you can adjust according to your personal needs without foregoing the basics.

After achieving your short term goal (let's say, lose weight), one of the best next goals in food combining is to attain a good disposition in life. This will prevent you from getting stressed, depressed, and therefore eating against your health.

There are many reasons why an average American woman should learn and practice proper food combining. The top of the list says that there is actually nothing to lose and everything to gain when you carefully monitor your diet. After all, as they commonly say, "you are what you eat". If you carelessly indulge in fatty, protein rich, sweet, and acidic foods, then your current personality shows that you do not care about your health. That being said, it is easy to say that you do not care about other people's health as well.

Our generation and the next generations need to know how to combine their foods correctly. Otherwise, they will go on believing that as long as they eat fruits and vegetables, and a good amount of carbs and protein, they will be fine.

No woman should suffer another day from weight gain, indigestion, inadequate supply of nutrients, and different types of avoidable and preventable illnesses. You can start as early as today and begin choosing the things you buy and eat in order to show how much you really care for your body (and for the environment and the whole human race as well!).

Bear in mind that food combining is an essential key to effective juicing. While it seems to be a whole separate complex idea that should be learned and practiced separately, food combining and juicing go well together and can be used to make each other more

fulfilling and bear more concrete results.

10. My Juicing Tip Sheet

There are so many fruits and vegetables to choose from. All of them are rich in vitamins, minerals and nutrients that cleanse your body and revitalize your life. But which ones do you really
need? Which combinations of nature's best produce would benefit you the most?

If you are at a loss for answers, no worries! This chapter is all about mastering your juicing menu with a personal juicing cheat sheet that lists down your choices and what good they do for your body. I have listed everything alphabetically and grouped them into fruits, vegetables (sea vegetables are also included), sprouts, nuts and herbs to make it as simple as possible.

Fruits

Fruits are naturally low in fat, sodium, on calories. They are also excellent sources of potassium, fiber, folic acid, vitamin C and other nutrients designed to make you better and stronger. While others will give words of caution about the sugar content of fruits, let us get one thing straight. Any fruit is better than none. And any fruit is far better than a piece of candy when your sweet tooth begins to crave. But if you are really worried about the sugar content, always strive for a variety of fruits and vegetables to make sure you get a good balance of nutrients.

Name of Fruit Why it is Good for You?

Apple- Apples are rich in vitamin C, iron, magnesium, phosphorus, magnesium and trace minerals. Juice this fruit for a natural immune boost. You also get a good dose of fiber that is good for the digestive tract.

Apricot- Apricots are low in fat, high in fiber, and rich in vitamins C B5, and E, potassium, and beta-carotene. Not only are apricots yummy, they are good for your eyes, your heart, and digestive tract.

Avocado- Avocados brim with leutein, potassium, protein, vitamin E, iron, and
good fats. They are delicious and versatile! Plus, avocados are rich in heart healthy monounsaturated fats and omega----three fatty acids. Good for the liver, and naturally lowers cholesterol. As a point of clarification, avocados are used for smoothies rather than juicing. But they do blend well with vegetable juices.

Bananas- Bananas are used for smoothies rather than juicing. Packed with potassium that protects the heart against high blood pressure and stroke. They are also a good source of iron, magnesium, vitamins B5 and B6, and vitamin C. Bananas help the heart, digestion, fat burn, and reduce risks for colorectal and kidney cancer.

Bell peppers- Bell peppers are usually classified as a vegetable, but this fruit is good for your heart, strengthens the immune system, protects against types of cancers, and oddly enough, fights sunburns. They are rich in beta----carotene, folate, vitamins C, B1, B2, B3, B5, B6, E and K, phytochemicals, and antioxidants.

Blackberry- Blackberries contain vitamins C, B5, E, K, beta-carotene,
phytonutrients, folate, iron, magnesium, and zinc. Blackberries fight free radicals in the body associated with heart disease and cancer. It also helps speed up fat burn.

Blueberry Called a super food because it is rich in antioxidants and phytonutrients, blueberries are also rich in vitamins C and K, fiber, manganese, and iron. Since they are loaded with vitamins, blueberries also help prevent illness and certain types of cancer.

Cantaloupe This fruit is a good source of beta-carotene, folate, potassium, and fiber. It also has high levels of vitamins C and B. Cantaloupes help prevent degenerative diseases that bog down the body, ideal for cleansing, rehydrating, and reducing inflammation.

Cherimoya A cherimoya tastes like a burst of strawberry, mango, and pineapple. It offers vitamins C, B1, B2, B3, B5, and B6, folate, iron, magnesium, phosphorus, potassium, omega----three fatty acids, and fiber. Cherimoyas are good for the heart and the brain. It also boosts immunity, prevents certain types of cancer, fights against osteoporosis, and Parkinson's disease.

Cherry Not everybody appreciates the tartness of cherry juice, but there is good reason to. Cherries are packed with nutrients such as vitamin C, magnesium, and iron. Because it is rich in antioxidants and anti----inflammatory agents, cherries promote body detoxification and boosts colon and heart health.

Cranberry Cranberry juice is an excellent source of vitamin C, oxalic acids, and dietary fiber. Those with urinary tract infections, respiratory disorders, kidney stones, heart disease and some types of cancer are prescribed to drink cranberry juice.

Cucumber Although some confuse cucumbers to be vegetables, they are actually fruit. They contain vitamins A, C, K and B5, calcium, potassium and iron. Cucumbers are good for your skin, hair, and nails. They aid in digestion and help prevent cancer. Plus, it promotes weight loss.

Dates Nutrient dense dates contain vitamins B5, B3, B2, beta-carotene, potassium, magnesium, phosphorus, calcium, iron, and fiber. Dates are good for the brain, heart and digestive health. They are also good for pregnancy.

Figs A good source of vitamins B1, B5, B6, beta-carotene, calcium,

manganese, iron, and calcium. Figs are low-calorie fruits that get high ratings from weight watchers. They are also a low-intensity laxative that is good for intestinal cleansing even for children.

Durian Despite the pungent smell, there is good reason to eat durian for its nutritional content. Durian is a good source of vitamins C, B1, B2, B3, B5, B6, folate, manganese, potassium, sulfur, magnesium, phosphorus, and iron. Durian has a warming effect on the body that is great for sleeping. It is also good for bone and digestive health, increased immunity, and cancer protection.

Grapefruit Grapefruit is rich in vitamins C, E, A, folate, niacin, pantothenic acid, pyridoxine, riboflavin, thiamin, potassium, calcium, iron, magnesium, phosphorus and zinc. Because the grapefruit is rich in nutrients, it makes the body stronger by protecting against heart disease and certain types of cancers. Plus, the fruit aids in weight loss.

Grapes contain health protecting antioxidants, including resveratrol and flavonoids. It also has a chockfull of nutrients such as Vitamins C, E, A, K, sodium, potassium, calcium, iron, magnesium, phosphorus and zinc. Grapes maintain healthy blood pressure and prevent certain cancers.

Jackfruits contain beta-carotene, vitamins C, B2 and B6. These fruits are good for digestive health and can also be used as a natural laxative.

Jujube   The jujube is rich in vitamin C, potassium, phosphorus, manganese, calcium, sodium, zinc, and iron. It boosts the immune system, lowers blood pressure; relieves stress and anxiety. It is also a natural sedative and has been known to cure some liver diseases.

Kiwi Kiwis have a delicious flavor and do the body good. Kiwis are packed with vitamins C, K, E, folate, iron, and potassium. They are excellent for digestion and skin health, and help remove excess sodium buildup.

Kumquat Kumquats look like small oval oranges. You eat it whole, including the skin. Kumquats have a high percentage of vitamin C, and a good source of calcium, beta-carotene and magnesium. They boost the immune system and helps fight against types of cancer.

Lemon   A lemon is rich in vitamins C, E, A; folate, niacin, pantothenic acid, pyridoxine, riboflavin and thiamin. It also contains sodium, potassium, calcium, iron, magnesium, phosphorus and zinc. Call it a super food if you will! Lemon juice stimulates the digestive tract, aids digestion, supports weight loss, promotes nerve and heart health, prevents kidney stones, and fights cancer.

Limes   Limes contain vitamin C, niacin, pantothenic acid, riboflavin and thiamin. It is also a good source of potassium, iron, magnesium and phosphorus. Limes help reverse the signs of aging and promote overall health. They are good for detox, as well as digestive, blood, nerve and heart health. Also good for cancer protection.

Longans Longans are a good source of vitamins A and C; iron, magnesium, phosphorus, and potassium. Longans are good for heart and blood health. They boost energy, and are also known to be good beauty and sex tonic. Always remember to remove the black pit before juicing.

Mangoes Good source of vitamin C, beta----carotene, calcium and potassium.
This fruit is good for renal, digestive and blood health. Also helps supports immune system.

Mangosteen Mangosteen is high in fiber, folate, and vitamins A and C. Many claim to have benefited from its antimicrobial and antiviral benefits. It helps protect against allergies, cancer, pain, high blood pressure, and inflammation.

Nectarines Nectarines are a rich source of beta----carotene, potassium, fiber, vitamins C, B3, and E. It contains antioxidants that help protect against cancer and other diseases by reducing cellular damage within the body.

Olives Olives are rich in monounsaturated fats, calcium, phosphorus, vitamins D and A. It also contains flavonoids and polyphenols that reduce inflammation in the body. It is good for those suffering from gastritis and ulcers; and helps prevent rickets and osteoarthritis.

Oranges Orange juice is the go----to drink for those in need of an immune boost. It contains one hundred seventy phytonutrients and more than sixty known falconoid. These two reduce inflammation, shrink tumors, and prevent blood clots. Oranges are also good in preventing cancers, heart problems, strokes, and constipation.

Papaya Papayas are extremely dense in beta----carotene, vitamin C, potassium, calcium, phosphorus, and iron. Juicing papaya brings many benefits.
It is good for the skin, for indigestion, constipation, irregular menstruation, and helps fight cancer.

Peaches In this fruit is a chockfull of vitamins C and A; lutein, lycopene, potassium, fiber, and niacin. Peaches are tough cancer fighters, it is also an antioxidant that protects against heart disease and macular degeneration.

Pear Pears have high content of vitamins C and E, as well as fiber, iodine, and copper. These make pears a source of powerful antioxidants that boost immunity and help prevent diseases such as cancer, high cholesterol, high blood pressure, and inflammatory conditions.

Pineapple Pineapples are loaded with vitamin C and various nutrients that help the body fight off disease, including cancer. They also contain a powerful enzyme called bromelain that acts as an inflammatory, aiding in the prevention of arthritis, swelling, carpal tunnel, gout, and sinusitis.

Plums Plums are a good source of fiber, oxalic acid, beta-carotene, antioxidants, phosphorus, potassium, as well as vitamins A, C, K, B6. Juicing plums can help the body with weight loss, iron absorption, smooth bowel movement, and strengthening the immune system.

Pomegranate Pomegranate juice is an excellent source of antioxidants like polyhpenols, tannins, and anthocyanins. Studies show that it fights prostate cancer and effective in lowering blood pressure. It is also good for the skin, urinary tract, and overall health.

Raspberries This fruit is high in vitamins C, K, A, and rich in potassium ellagic acid, magnesium, and phosphorus. Because of its high nutrient content, it is known to lower cholesterol, slow down cancer, and prevent cardiovascular problems.

Strawberry Strawberries are rich in vitamin C, folate, potassium, vitamins, and minerals. They are known to protect against Alzheimer's disease, reduce bad cholesterol, and prevent certain types of cancers. Strawberries also relieves sore muscles and stress.

Tangerine Tangerines help you hydrate because of its high water content. High amounts of vitamins A and C boost the immune system and help fight infections. They also provide the body with beta-carotene, calcium, magnesium, and potassium.

Tomato Apart from being rich in vitamins C, K, B1, B5, and B6, tomatoes contain a powerful antioxidant called lycopene, which protects the liver, lungs, prostate gland, skin, and colon. Scientific studies about lycopene show that it helps prevent macular degeneration, lowers cholesterol, and prevents cancer.

Watermelon Naturally----packed with vitamin C, beta----carotene, riboflavin, niacin, potassium, sodium, zinc, lycopene and a bunch of other nutrients. These help you stay healthy while reducing the risk of ovarian and cervical cancer. It also helps you shed extra pounds.

Vegetables

Vegetables are packed with enzymes, nutrients, vitamins, and minerals crucial to overall health and wellbeing. Juicing is a great way to get these nutrients into your body, and an excellent means of getting your recommended dose of vegetable servings each day.

Name of Vegetable Why it is Good for You?

Asparagus Contains vitamins C, B1, B2, and B3, plus beta----carotene, folic acid, and fiber. It is a natural diuretic and laxative, good for the heart, and great for the kidneys.

Beets Your digestive system and kidneys will thank you for consuming beets. It has copper, magnesium, iron, potassium, and manganese.

Bok Choy Rich in antioxidants, vitamins A and C, beta----carotene, calcium, and fiber.

Broccoli Known as a super food! It is nutrient----dense and protects against types of cancer, promotes healthy vision, and helps body detox.

Cabbage Its high fiber content aids in digestion. It also has yttrium and selenium that cleanses the mucous membrane of the stomach and intestinal tract.

Carrot Carrots are excellent sources of beta----carotene, potassium, and selenium. They help eye function, infections, improve liver function, and help protect against cancer.

Cauliflower They are nutrient----dense and full of antioxidants. As a tip though, juice the base and not the florets.

Celery Celery is high in organic sodium, magnesium, and iron that help cleanse the digestive system of uric acid. It also has vitamin C that helps in cancer prevention.

Chlorella Though it is an algae, it is considered a super food. It is anti----cancer and good for detoxification.

Collards Collards are rich in chlorophyll, antioxidants, and other nutrients. It also has good amounts of vitamins C, K, B1, B2, B3, B5, and B6. Collard greens protect against hemorrhoids and colon cancer.

Corn Yes, corn can be juiced. Just be careful to choose organic corn and avoid genetically modified ones. Corn has vitamins C, B1, B2, B3, B5, and B6, as well as other good----for----you nutrients. Not too much though as it is high in sugar.

Dandelion The bitter dandelion greens are excellent blood cleansers, detoxifiers, and digestive aid. They are a source of vitamins C, B1, B2, B6, K and

E, beta-carotene, folate, calcium, fiber, sodium, and omega six.

Kale Some also call kale a super food as it is an excellent source of chlorophyll, calcium, iron, sulfur, beta-carotene, and a chockfull of vitamins. It fights inflammation, prevents cancer, and helps the body detox.

Kelp Kelp is high in minerals, folate, iron, calcium, zinc, sodium, phosphorus, copper, and vitamins K and E.

Lettuce Dark green varieties of lettuce (and not iceberg lettuce) are a good source of chlorophyll. It is mostly water and contains vitamins, folate, potassium, iron, calcium and other nutrients.

Nori You should add nori or laver to your juicing list as it is nutrient and vitamin dense. It boosts immunity with high content of beta-carotene and vitamins C, B1, B2, B3, B5, B6, and E.

Okra Okra soothes the digestive tract by coating the intestines and acting as a natural lubricant. It is good for people with digestion problems, but do not use more than one okra per quart or it can change the consistency of your juice.

Onions Onions are natural detoxifiers, antiseptics, and stimulants. Add a little bit of onion into your juice from time to time to reap the rewards of its nutrient----dense contents.

Parsnip Parsnips are a great source of folate, fiber, manganese, copper, and vitamins C, E, B1, and B5. They are known to detox and cleanse the body.

Peas Peas can go into your juice too! They add protein, vitamins, minerals, and nutrients into your concoction.

Peppers Peppers can boost the metabolism, making it a great fat----burner. They also contain beta-carotene, vitamins C and B6, copper, iron, manganese, magnesium, and omega six.

Pumpkin Pumpkins reduce inflammation. They also lower risks for lung and prostate cancer. Plus, they are a good source of beta----carotene, vitamins B2, C, and E, copper, iron, and potassium.

Radish Those with thyroid, liver, and stomach problems will benefit from radish. They also aid in weight loss by adding to the feeling of fullness. Radish has a generous amount of folate, vitamin C, copper, iron, and zinc.

Spinach Spinach is very dense in nutrients. It is good for the blood because of its iron and chlorophyll content. It is also rich in vitamins B2 and B6, minerals, iron, and potassium.

Squash Winter squash is great for the eyes and heart. It is a cancer----fighter because of its high beta-carotene content. It is also dense in vitamins B1, B5, B6, and C, copper, iron, magnesium, manganese, phosphorus, and potassium.

Sweet potato Sweet potatoes are natural detoxifiers, support digestion, anti----cancer, and good for the body. They contain beta----carotene, vitamins B1, B5, B6, copper, iron, magnesium, manganese, phosphorus, and potassium.

Turnip   Turnips help fight cancer and are known for anti----biotic and anti----viral benefits. The bottom line is that they make your body stronger.

Zucchini Good to eat, good to juice. Has vitamins C, B, A; lutein, folate, and potassium.

Nuts
Milk from nuts has become a popular substitute for health enthusiasts. It is lactose----free and packed with nutrients.
While making milk from nuts will not really go with your juice, you can use them as a base for smoothies. You can also add some nuts on top of your juice for texture and flavor.

Almonds Almond milk is high in protein, potassium, magnesium, phosphorus, and calcium.

Chestnut Chestnut milk is low in fat, contains complete B vitamins, and an excellent source of fiber.

Cashew Cashew milk is high in protein, vitamin A, potassium, and magnesium.

Coconut Coconut milk is a great source of electrolytes, copper, iron, magnesium, manganese, phosphorus, potassium, zinc, iodine, and selenium.

Hazel Hazelnut milk is delicious and high in protein, calcium, potassium, and sulfur.

Pecans Pecan milk is good for the heart, with ample amounts of protein, potassium, and vitamin A.

Walnuts Walnut milk is also rich in protein, magnesium, vitamin A, and magnesium.

11. Detox Juicing

Detox juicing benefits the body by eliminating toxins that weaken the immune system and make us prone to degenerative diseases. This chapter aims to answer the why's and how's of detox juicing, and tips on how to kick start your own detox.

What Toxins Are You Talking About?

We live in a society consumed by fast food, processed foods, and artificially flavored drinks. It seems as though the grit and grind of hectic everyday life has caught up to our bodies. In giving our bodies nutrition from the fastest and easiest sources possible, we have made difficult to pronounce chemicals a staple of our everyday diet. These toxins hamper our body's natural ability to balance sugar and metabolize cholesterol. And as we continue to consume them, we turn our bodies into a breeding ground of fat and disease.

A 2009 report by the Centers for Disease Control and Prevention (CDC) on human exposure to environmental chemicals revealed that every person the CDC tested had a host of chemicals inside their body. Shocking, right? This list of toxic cocktails included chemicals from flame retardants and a hormone like substance called Bisphenol A (2) found in plastic. Even more shocking was the finding that the average newborn has almost three hundred chemicals found in the umbilical cord. Below are some of the more common toxins, preservatives, and additives we consume everyday:

Pesticides

Have you heard of the dirty dozen? Apples, celery, peaches, sweet bell peppers, nectarines, strawberries, cherries, pears, grapes, spinach, lettuce, and potatoes are known to have high amounts of pesticides. Choosing organic alternatives to these twelve can reduce your exposure to pesticides by eighty percent.

Pesticides accumulate in our bodies over time. Our bodies cannot remove them even if they do damage to our endocrine, reproductive, circulatory, immune, and central nervous systems. A recent study showed that all of us have dangerous traces of polychlorinated biphenyls (PCBs), dioxin, chlordane, aldrin, dieldrin, and dioxin in our blood streams. Scary!

Sodium nitrate and nitrite

If you love processed foods and meat products, then you expose yourself regularly to sodium nitrate and nitrite. Yes, hotdogs, ham, corned beef, luncheon meat, and many others belong to this list.

Caffeine

Natural caffeine in moderation is fine. But too much (especially if it comes from gum, soda, diet soda, and the link) is addictive, affects fertility, and is even known to cause birth defects, heart conditions, behavioral changes, osteoporosis, and insomnia.

BHA/BHT

If you have the habit of reusing or reheating oil to save a few bucks stop! Oil that is used again has BHA/BHT that increases appetite, affects sleep, and causes problems to the liver, kidney, heart, and even cancer. Throw old oil away!

Refined Sugar

Never has the world consumed so much candy through sweets, candies, chocolates, cakes name it! However, this toxic love affair leads to diabetes, weight gain, arthritis, migraines, decreased immunity, gallstones, breast cancer, and heart disease. In fact, many diseases can be linked to too much sugar.

Sugar Sweetened Drinks

Artificial sweeteners like saccharin, aspartame, and NutraSweet affect brain neurochemistry. These are found in soft drinks, sport drinks, and other sweetened beverages.

Monosodium Glutamate or MSG

MSG is not just found in food, even candy, gums, and yogurt has trace amounts of it. MSG is harmful because it causes obesity and inhibits our natural growth hormone. It also causes headaches, nausea, weakness, and changes in heart rate.

Brominated Vegetable Oil (BVO) and Partially Hydrogenated Vegetable Oil

These two reduce immunity, increase allergic reactions, elevate cholesterol levels, and has even been tied to certain types of cancer. BVO is toxic to children, while Partially Hydrogenated Vegetable Oil is full of trans fat making it toxic to adults.

Now that you have an idea of the toxins consumed everyday, does it not seem like the world is caught up in a vicious toxic cycle? If you are ready to cleanse and give your body a fighting chance against an unhealthy lifestyle, then get your juicer ready and reap the benefits of detox juicing.

Benefits Of Detox Juicing

The human body is so amazing that it has the ability to cleanse itself of most toxins we consume. We can thank the liver and the kidneys for that. However, with the amount of toxins we are ingesting, detox juicing can step in to combat the effects of an unhealthy way of eating and living. Here are three of its top benefits:

1. Detox juicing means subsisting on pressed juices from fruits and vegetables for a few days. As we know, fruits and vegetables are nutrient dense! It is an excellent way to get more phytonutrients from vegetables and fruits into your body.

Juicing allows you to absorb the nutrients with less digestive work required.

2. It can help you jumpstart a healthy new routine.
3. It eliminates fats, sugar, and processed foods from the diet. Indeed, detox juicing can result in increased energy, clearer skin, and less digestive issues.

As a general and wisdom filled rule, it is always best to consult your physician before entering any new regimen. And be sure to check that your juicing program gives you all the nutrients calories you need per day.

Getting Started

Juicing provides us with a simple yet satisfying way to end unhealthy eating and reset our metabolism. But before you begin, there are eleven important points to take into consideration.

First, know why you want to do detox juicing.

Your primary motivation must be your own physical wellbeing and flushing out toxins from your system. Do not do it because your friends said so, or because your favorite celebrity endorsed it.

Also, it is no secret that everyone wants to lose extra pounds. But do not make weight loss the moving force behind your juice detox. Fruits can be high in sugar, so you may feel disappointed if you do not get the weight loss results you hoped for. Weight loss follows naturally after you become committed to living and eating clean.

Choose a juice detox program that is right for you.

The standard detox regimen will take two to four days, but a longer detox will have the most beneficial outcome. As mentioned earlier, choose a program that will provide enough nutrients and calories for you to exist without headaches and low morale. In other words, choose a program you know you can stick to! There is nothing worse than binging on a toxic buffet because your four day juice detox has left you too hungry.

Prepare yourself physically and mentally.

Detoxification is an important and necessary step prior to any program. It is the time to wean yourself from unhealthy habits. For many years, toxins, preservatives, chemicals, and caffeine have found a happy home in our system causing addiction. Think of them like narcotics and nicotine—they are hard to let go of, and if you do find the strength to break free, you should prepare for withdrawal systems.

Give yourself three to five days to prepare for your upcoming detox. This is the usual time people can adjust to changes into their lifestyle and diet. Start by making a list of habits that are causing harm to your body and gradually limit your indulgence of them. A word of caution though—some people get terrible migraines, cramps, or even fall into depression from keeping away the things that they think make their day complete. It could be cigarettes, too much coffee, chips, or chocolate!

Start taking in a lot of fresh fruits and vegetables to ease yourself into the pre----detox process. For example, instead of taking coffee, eggs, and bacon for breakfast, a fresh glass of grapefruit or orange juice and an apple in the morning is a great start. Limit also the amount of fat intake by eating salads with lemon juice and herbs with daily meals cutting down on the amount of fatty or processed foods. Even eating half of your normal daily intake can do wonders.

Plan out your detox.

The first two days on a juice detox will be the hardest. Your body will adjust—and it might even rebel a bit. That is why it is better to start on a Thursday or Friday and continue over the weekend when your workload is low.

Get your goods ready.

Freshness is important when doing detox juicing. Unlike cooking that eliminates a lot of important vitamins and minerals naturally found in fresh fruits and vegetables, juicing lets you take nutrients in quickly and effectively.

One day before your detox, head to the farmer's market or the grocery to buy your fruits and vegetables. Buy the freshest ingredients and avoid canned produce. If you have the time, it is always advisable to buy your fruit and vegetables a day prior to use so you can get the optimum nutrient content. Buying organically grown produce will also ensure that you do not ingest any of the pesticides you are trying to rid your body of. Once you get them home and you are not sure they are organic, do a quick rinse of water with a small amount of vinegar or lemon juice to do the trick.

Detox juicing is a simple and easy way to detoxifying or cleansing yourself. There is no need for elaborate preparations, you simply choose which of nature's gifts to drink today and pop them into your juicer. Preparation time is fast because all you need is a good juicer and a good knife (to cut the large pieces of fruit or vegetables), and you are ready to go. Cut, juice, and drink.

Drink the right amount of juice.

When doing a juicing cleanse, it is recommended that you drink anywhere from thirty two to ninety six fluid ounces of juice per day to get the optimal cleansing effect. And drink lukewarm water in between juice intake to help with absorption and toxin elimination. Remember, water is your friend, especially during your juice detox.

Here is an example of how a basic detox juicing regiment might go:

• When you wake up in the morning, drink lukewarm water infused with lemon and cucumbers. This can be prepared the night before.
• A glass of cashew or almond milk.
• Take between eight to twenty four ounces of juice, four times within the day that includes three servings of green vegetable juice – mix of spinach, kale, celery stalks, romaine lettuce, cucumber with some apple and lemon to taste. Also include one serving of beets, carrot and apple juice within the day.
•   End with a glass of cashew or almond milk.

You will start to feel the effects two to three days after you start. And you will feel a whole lot better once the cleansing is done.

The days after your juice cleanse are just as crucial. You should begin slowly re introducing different foods to your diet. Do this slowly and listen to your body after each intake of food. If a certain food makes you feel sick, it means your body is reacting to. Since cleansing has eliminated the toxins, your body will let you know loud and clear if something does not agree with you.

Stay hydrated.

It is common knowledge that we should drink a lot of water daily. It has so many benefits that you should drink six to eight glasses per day regardless if you are cleansing or not. Water energizes muscles, maintains fluid balance in the bodies, helps our kidneys, and essential for overall health. Plus, it has no preservatives or additives. It is one hundred percent good for the body. Water is vital to the cleansing process. Drinking a lot of water will help speed up detoxification and will help your body burn fat. It also helps give the feeling of fullness should you get hunger pangs.

Get enough sleep.

When changing one's lifestyle, it is important to get at least eight hours of sleep daily. Some may get by with six hours of rest, but eight will get you the best results. Without proper rest, one may become stressed and mentally exhausted. Stress is a major hindrance during the detoxification process. A lack of sleep can lead to headaches, nausea, and decrease in energy. And while you are set on getting enough hours of sleep, be sure to turn in early as well. Studies show that sleeping before eleven in the evening is optimal for the body to rejuvenate and heal itself.

Are you finding it hard to sleep? Try breathing exercises and meditation to relax your body and wind down.

Conserve energy.

The first few days of a juice detox will be met by challenges. You might feel a bit weak as your body adjusts to your juice intake. That is why most are advised to limit their exercise and training program during the detox regimen. It will only be for a few days anyway, and the benefits of the juice cleanse far outweigh the burden of skipping the gym for two to four days.

Too much strenuous activity can have an adverse effect on you. Your body is scrambling for energy during your detox phase, so if you push it by keeping the intensity level high during your workout you may only be doing yourself more harm than good.

There are acceptable forms of exercise during the detox period: a brisk walk or a light swim is perfectly fine. You can use this alone time to relax and meditate. Massages and other relaxing activities are also encouraged during your cleanse. Remember that being relaxed and rested will boost your body's detox process.

Have a support group.

One of the best ways to succeed in a juice cleanse is to surround yourself with positive and supportive people. A detox buddy or a support group is highly recommended. It could be a family member or a friend who could be doing the same detox program as you are.

Accountability is a big word! It means that you own up to your actions and that you are taking responsibility for your decisions! Having a support group helps you strengthen your resolve to be accountable to your body. Your buddy is there to give you a needed push when you hit a wall and you feel like giving up.

If there is no one you know who could be a support buddy at this time, why not go online and join a health forum? You would be surprised to find how many people are going through the same experience as you are facing now.

Juice-on-the-go.

If you are a person who is always on the go, you can still do a detox juicing. It will just take extra preparation and making your juice in advanced. Invest in a few BPA----free containers and prepare all your ingredients the night before. Juice your produce in the morning. Ideally, you should consume your juice within one hour from the time you made them. But you can also bring around a cooler with a lot of ice to keep your juice chilled and fresh. Some have even bought portable juicers and made their health tonics right in the office pantry. Yes, it can be done!

Detox juicing is about giving back to your self. Ultimately, you decide to go on a juice cleanse because you want to do your body good. And with all the benefits of detox juicing,

this method is a great way to take back your health and jumpstart a clean and
nutrient rich lifestyle!

12. Conclusion

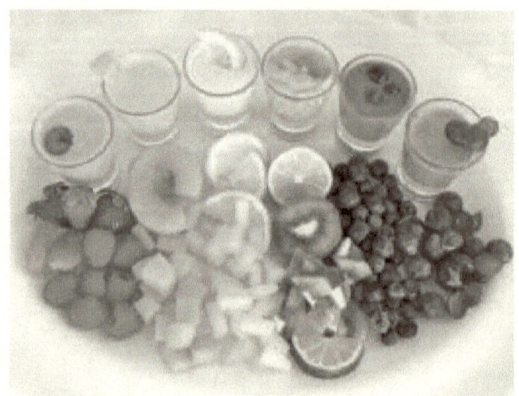

We live in a world consumed by a diet of fat, processed foods, preservatives, and countless toxic substances. Scientific research is showing that majority of people have an internal cocktail of toxic chemicals that confuse our body, result in imbalance, and lead to an
array of chronic diseases. Come to think of it, there has never been a time when the incidences of obesity, cancer, and cardiovascular disease have become so rampant.

If there is one thing we have learned, it is that cure and prevention is within reach. We simply have to look at fruits, vegetables, herbs, nuts, and seeds to provide us with potent nutrients and anti-oxidants that can build the foundation of a strong and healthy life. Every trip to the market and the grocery can become your health revolution. And all you need is your juicer to get started!

If you have picked up this book, it means you are ready to take back your health and heal yourself through natural alternatives. And with the knowledge the past thirteen chapters have shared with you, I am sure you are now well on your way to being a pro in juicing fresh fruits and vegetables!

Juices pressed from fruits and vegetables are not only delicious, they are super healthy. In its juice form, vitamins and minerals are easily digested and absorbed, allowing our bodies to maximize the nutrients and antioxidants nature meant for us to receive. And much more, they are effective fighters of the common diseases we have today due to an unhealthy lifestyle.

So what are you waiting for? Ready, press, juice!

13. THANK YOU FOR READING !

Thank You so much for reading this book. If this title gave you a ton of value, It would be amazing for you to leave a REVIEW !

THANK YOU FOR DOWNLOADING! IF YOU ENJOYED THIS BOOK AND WOULD LIKE TO READ MORE TITLES FROM MY COLLECTION CLICK THIS LINK